MW01168518

Medical Intuition
Intuitive Diagnosis

MIDI-Medical Intuitive Diagnostic Imaging™
and
AMIDI- Animal Medical Intuitive Diagnostic Imaging™

Learn how to see inside a body to interpret the bioenergy
patterns that identify and diagnose
past, current and future diseases and disorders.

Brent Atwater

Just Plain Love® Books

inspiring thoughts that provide smiles, hugs and healing
for every reader's heart!

This *Just Plain Love*® Book
is given

To: _____

Message: _____

_____

with
LOTS of LOVE
and
HUGS!!!

From: _____

Date: _____

                Library of Congress Cataloging-in-Publication Data

                Paperback ISBN-13: 978-1439274101
                        ISBN-10: 143927410X
                        Hardcover ISBN:
                        EBook ISBN:
                Kindle ASIN: B0043M6LCC
                    2nd printing: 2011 USA
                            Canada
UK, AU, SA check with distributor Publisher's Price Higher in Other Countries

Christian/ Protestantism Holistic Healthcare/ Self Development Lifestyles / Self-
Help/ Spiritual Growth / Mind Body Connection / Energy Medicine / Alternative
Healthcare / Holistic Medicine / Self Development Intuitive Healing / Spirituality
/ Integrated Medicine / Law of Attraction/ Religion & Spirituality / Christianity /
Protestantism Body, Mind & Spirit medicine/ Self Healing / Nonfiction / Audio
Books / eBooks / Kindle

Acknowledgements

I want to thank all of those who have supported
and encouraged my journey;
and the authors, speakers and teachers who
contributed to shaping my consciousness and continuing education.

Special thanks to Michael Wellford,
and my beloved pets for their contributions
and enduring patience with my spiritual path.

My greatest gratitude goes to my first client Hank, and all others that
followed, my friends and family members who allowed me to
"look at" their health "experience" and the opportunity to experience
viewing their body's theater which created the inspiration and
substance for this book.

I am also grateful for Dr. Larry Burk and
Dr. Laurance Johnston's guidance and support. Thanks to
Vanna Virata for her insights for this book, to
Dr. Leon Curry for providing invaluable insight, suggestions &
encouragement for my book.
Thanks to Nancie Benson for her expansive analytical questions.

A special thanks to Meg Post for her inexhaustible supply of patience
and attention to details,
and to
Maude or Myrtle for their support and tenaciousness.
Also to Catherine with a C and Mr. Magic Garvin for
all their "get it done right!" help for this and all my books!
***
I also want to thank you the reader for taking your time to explore my
Just Plain Love® Books and for allowing me to share what I have
learned and am learning.
It is my intent is that each book inspires thoughts that provide smiles,
hugs and healing for every reader's heart.

It is my hope and intent that this information will help you have
insight, greater perspectives, expanded awareness and knowledge.

Dedication

I write this book to honor and give thanks for the wonderful Gift
that I have the privilege of being the steward of,
and the opportunity to serve and share with others.

To all those inspiring and courageous individuals
with whom I shared and share their healing journey
and experiences and
who provided the literal body "insight"
to produce this book.

To Thomas Michael Ramseur Wellford,
whose life, love, and passing
made my understanding possible.
I shall always hold you and hear you
in my heart, my soul, and my dreams.

To those very special people and pets
who have been and are my joy,
with whom I have shared and share hope, laughter and LIFE!!!

Special Gratitude

to all my "voices" and guides and the other energies and entities who
serve the Christ White Light named and unnamed who were relentless,
impatient, persistent, exhausting, exasperating, informative, accurate,
edgy, humorous, entertaining, deliberate, persuasive, detailed beyond
belief and always of the highest integrity and utmost determination for
me and my clients' highest and best good.
I admire their patience with my path, their directives for my education
and evolution and their ongoing and forever
training of my soul.
They are my best friends, greatest teachers, constant companions,
best protectors, collaborators, and support team.
Namaste! Et al Y'all ☺

Table of Contents

*Everything you ever need to learn, see or know
resides inside of you!*

*Part 1
Your job is to choose, accept, trust, protect,
cleanse and allow the Gift to flow through you*

Part 2
Show up with accountability, responsibility,
and integrity.

Part 3
*Trust the information given to you
by your Higher Power and Guides.*

Part 4
*Detach remove and release from your client
and session. Go onto your next experience
unfettered and unaffected by energy, issues or entities.*

Part 5
Go home and enjoy your life on earth!

Introduction

I love the science of medical intuitive diagnosis! I love looking into each client's body. To me, each body is a wonderful theater providing a unique view of each and every play in all the stages of an individual's life!

The body is awesome. I'm amazed at what it can do, how it functions, how it regenerates, and how it readapts to life altering situations right before my eyes.

I approach every new experience with accountability, humility and appreciation in addition to the blessed responsibility of my Gift.

However, seeing medical disorders and disease so graphically within each human or animal's life sometimes takes a momentary toll on my heart. I have to focus on the fact that my Gift is to benefit others and remember how it helps their lives with accurate insight, relative information and intuitive directives that facilitate each soul's healing journey.

Sitting in North Carolina literally looking at the cancer ridden intestinal sac of a woman in the Philippines that I have never met and just spoken with for about 5 minutes, or viewing the disconnected cranial nerve in a client's brain in Greece that is causing her double vision and seizures is an awesome experience.

Watching the heartbeat monitor of a child stabilize under my directive gaze thousands of miles away, or having a client report the bleeding is stopping, the respiration rate is steadied or the oxygen levels are raising more than half way around the world is proof to me there is a Higher Power! Even knowing when a nurse is moving your patient (located across the across the globe) or administering a treatment proves you're "in touch" with their energy field and creates humility!

All of the above, to me, is proof of a Higher Power's omnipotent presence, knowledge and participation in the greater good.

When I lie down in an MRI, I watch and monitor the exact same images the MRI machine is documenting on film and transmitting to the technicians. It's fascinating and a bit unnerving.
My friends laugh and say the MRI is my Mother!

I KNOW there is a God and a Universal Higher Power and connection when I actually see, understand, evaluate, assess and diagnose a human's energy and physical anatomy with astounding accuracy and incredible detail, especially since I have had no medical training to color or prejudice my opinions or affect my findings.

I offer my experience and medical intuitive diagnostic imaging™ (MIDI) bioenergy patterns and codes to each holistic integrative energy medicine professional, intuitive healer, educator, researcher, medical intuitive student, dreamer and curious reader from my soul's "experiences" during sickness, degenerating health, disease, chronic illness and even sudden or inevitable death.

I have been the patient, caregiver, friend, instructor, cheerleader, medical intuitive, energy healer, consultant, and bearer of good and bad tidings. I've supported those who were dying and helped in their transition. I have shared disorders, disabilities, despair, untimely death, miracles, healing and triumphant joy personally and with my clients.

Many thanks to all those who have taught me what I share with you. I can only activate within you, facilitate, teach and empower your innate skills to the level that God has intended your soul to experience in this lifetime.

Do not be discouraged if you cannot do exactly what my Gifts accomplish. My Gifts were created for my individual contributions.

You are created uniquely to perform what YOU came to contribute which is not one iota less or more important than anyone else. We all serve humanity with our different skills and Gifts.

Everything that I present in this books will not interfere with what you do or with any intuitive or healing modalities. These tools and techniques will most likely enhance, amplify, awaken, inspire and ignite and expand your current abilities.

Use only that information which resonates with your soul.

Definitions

I'm setting forth the definitions for the verbiage that I use in this book so we'll be on the "same page" to more clearly understand what I am trying to communicate.

Every client is a master teacher for me to learn the energy language and images of the body. Since this energy language has so many visual images that are symbolic for diseases, disorders, medical conditions and health issues, I felt it needed to be shared. We each have our symbolism; however, it is my intent that the bioenergy patterns from my MIDI method of medical intuitive diagnostic imagining™ will give you a better and more thorough understanding of what you perceive. I hope it will expand your awareness and accuracy to deductively interpret and diagnose what you see.

The reason I assign colors to each image is the fact that each color corresponds to a specific electromagnetic vibrational frequency. In Roslyn Bruyere's *Wheels of Light*, she notes that each color has a measurable frequency that corresponds to energy. You'll find a lot of information in her book.

Active areas are active health disorder issues in current energy.

Clairaudience "is receiving messages in thought form from another frequency or realm in a normal state of consciousness. It is considered a form of channeling. It is the ability to hear things not audible within normal hearing ranges. Clairaudience may refer not to actual perception of sound, but may instead indicate impressions of the "inner mental ear" similar to the way many people think words without having auditory impressions. But it may also refer to actual perception of sounds such as voices, tones, or noises which are not apparent to other humans or to recording equipment."
The intuitive may be "told" about issues through their Guides and Universal helpers.

Clair cognizance means clear knowing. A claircognizant knows, without knowing how he knows. According to Doreen Virtue that's how "Divine wisdom enters our mind to serve the world."

Clairsentience is the ability to feel and capture information through sensations or "clear feeling."
"Clairsentients receive a lot of guidance through their intuition, gut feelings, and hunches and messages through their heart, emotions and physical reactions." Being an empath although informative is not healthy for the intuitive as it can wreak havoc with the reader's energy field. If you are a medical intuitive and an empath, shield yourself from other people's energy and ask to know the information in another way.

Clairvoyance is a noun from late 17th century French [Clair (clear) & voyant (seeing)] and is defined as a "form of extra-sensory perception". Clairvoyance "is the art of 'seeing' with senses beyond the five. Clairvoyance is often called the 'sixth sense' or ESP. It is the psychic ability or power to see objects, and visions, or to gain information regardless of its distance. The visions may also be in the future, and some times in the past. Clairvoyance is an umbrella term which often refers to telepathy, spiritualism, psychic research, second sight, prophetic visions, and dreams."

FYI "ESP" Extra Sensory Perception is an "umbrella term" that includes all the "paranormal" modalities that psychics and medical intuitives receive such as those mentioned above. ESP also includes the sense of "just knowing." According to Leon E. Curry, M.D. a pioneer in the scientific study of psychic medical diagnosis by medical intuition (see his book *The Doctor and the Psychic*) "those modalities seem to 'mimic' information received by our more 'normal' receptor organs. The receptors of ESP information have not yet been identified as to their location or how they work in contrast to our "normal" receptors (eyes, etc.) We do know gifted individuals do receive information paranormally as has been proven scientifically over and over since Dr. J. B. Rhine's experiments in the 1930's."

Emotional Scan reviews the current energy field of all feelings and is commonly called the heart's energy. It relates to all present and past emotional issues that are contained in an energy field.

Future energy is the last outermost energy overlay on a body's energy field. Health issues can possibly be corrected by a client's choices before they manifest into the body's energy if addressed by medication and or life choices.

Example, even though I see a future cancer metastasis, chemotherapy, radiation treatments or alternative therapy treatments may arrest its future development into the physical energy.

Physical Body Scan known in the traditional medical field as an intuitive anatomical medical diagnosis addresses your current physical energy although everything that has happened to your body is held in your cellular memory blueprint.

A reputable medical intuitive will be able to separate the old physical energy from your current issues and possibly be able to read your future health issue energy patterns that can occur. This scan evaluates the vibrational frequencies in your various physical systems: cells, organs, bones, tissue, etc.

FYI, a healthy body resonates at 68-72 MHz. You can find the body's organs vibrational frequencies on the Internet.

Brent Atwater's *Just Plain Love® Books* presents
MIDI- How to See Inside a Body to Identify & Intuitively Diagnose Disorders

20

the Journey Begins

The phone rings and a client halfway across the globe, asks to speak to Brent Atwater Medical Intuitive. I say "this is she." Oftentimes the client is taken aback that sometimes I answer my office's phone. I presume they would like to speak with the person they want to work with.

The client asks if I can evaluate what their physicians have not ascertained and if I can provide suggestions. I state that I can look into their body at the organs, blood, tissues bones, brain, vascular and pulmonary systems, nerves and all the other "insides" and tell them what I see.

With that visual information I can intuitively tell them what, where, how intense and answer other questions relating to what I find. Then I can suggest what tests to take, where to tell their healthcare professionals to look, and I furnish medical words so they can discuss these concepts or areas with their doctor. Additionally I relate that we can look at the energy as it presents for future prognosis.

My visual span is from prebirth up to the present and into the future. Every individual's energy contains a timeline that I can follow and "track," interpret and diagnose.

For a split second at the end of each call, I remember all that has happened beforehand to allow me to have my Gift's incredible journey.

I'm presenting this book's contents in the order that I learned each step along the way. Perhaps it will seem familiar to you and your journey, make your awakening less frightening and more awesome, or illuminate a place within yourself that is vaguely familiar or provide expanded awareness for those seeking to enlarge their knowledge base. Perhaps it will ignite all that you are and can be, or at least provoke some interesting thoughts and questions within your mind.

I was in the original Extra Sensory Perceptions (ESP) group tested by Dr. J. B. Rhine from Duke University at age 5. His research team study documented that I had a 98% receivership ability and a 97% sending ability (at least that's what they told me). Like I knew what that meant!

I did know that I loved the days when "the men in the white lab coats" would come and play mind games with me and my other classmates in another building. We played guess the dominos and number sequences, or what our classmates were doing or what they were writing (while located in another building) that they wanted to tell me. It was fun.

When I went to college, I was asked who I went to school with by my girlfriends and I stated "the same people that I stared first grade with." My classmates, said "why?" I thought that was normal.

Later I discovered that our school system had been picked to sequester this particular group of children that had been tested and received mental testing scores that were considered "Gifted" for the initial test run of Governor Terry Sanford's "Gifted Program" in the school's grade 1 -12 system. Later our project would become the pilot program that provided all the guidelines for the national "Gifted programs" in 1-12 education.

The teachers throughout our various grades taught us a lot of interesting things. One of the most fascinating concepts was introduced in our freshman year. We were told that due to our mental prowess, several of us might not be able to handle all of our sensory input and might choose to leave. (Earth)
So we were taught how to disconnect and cut off our mind's chatter or excessive input so it wouldn't disrupt our daily lives.

Later in college, several of my most brilliant classmates did commit suicide. After that occurred I mastered how to shut off my thoughts when I wanted to do so and practiced it regularly!

As I maneuvered through life, I thought that seeing energy was just normal and listening to my intuition about everything was also normal. Example, at one point after purchasing a new home, when I would come near the toilet I'd hear the word "septic tank."
The only way to ever cease my inner guidance is to do something about the subject matter. So I called a company, explained that I had just moved into a new home and knew nothing about septic tanks. I asked would they please send someone out to check the septic system.

As soon as the man completed his work, he informed me "Lady, if you had not called us today, your septic system's contents would have backend up into your bathtub and all your sinks."
THANK YOU inner guidance! I NEVER discount and always act on the advice that I am given even regarding septic tanks!

In 1997 my beloved best friend and fiancé Michael Wellford was killed in an unexpected automobile crash. Several days after his death, ALL my Gifts exploded full front and center and were driving me crazy.

Regress for a moment. Actually the Gift started before Mike left on Easter Sunday. The last thing I said to him was "Mikey, please don't drive down here next weekend, you are so tired you're gonna kill yourself in that car!" Little did I know my inner guidance was giving me a "heads up."

I had talked to Mike on the phone at 6:30 pm and he said he would be arriving at 9:30 pm. At 9:30 I was having excruciating pains in my chest to the point of calling a friend and asking her to keep talking to me until Mike arrived in case I needed to go to the emergency room. About 9:45, the pain subsided and I got off the phone and said I'll just wait till Mike arrives any minute now.

Unbeknownst to me, Mike had fallen asleep at the wheel and was in a car wreck around 9:30. The steering wheel went through his chest and he died about 9:45.

After the funeral I went to Duke University Medical Center and sat in the waiting room determined to meet the head of the Integrative Medical Center. A man popped his head around a corner after hour 6.5 and asked who I wanted to see. After I told him, he stated, "I am Dr. Larry Burk, you are looking for me!"

I told him what was happening. He immediately took me into a freshman class of his x-ray students and asked me what was wrong with each person's x-ray displayed on the room's huge wall monitors. Information just spilled out of me like I knew what I was doing. I didn't. I had no medical education or degree as I majored in creative writing and art at Hollins University and then attended Wake Forest University Law School.

Of note: Prior to this occurring, my friends always thought it was funny that I was mesmerized by the *New England Journal of Medicine* and the *Journal of the American Medical Association*, *Prevention* and any and all other health informative magazines were my favorite things to read for leisure. You'll learn later that inexplicable deep seated interests like this are known to your soul; even though these interests are not in flow with the life you are currently living (I was modeling in New York.)

Dr. Burk sent me home with a list of books to read, and told me I was a "medical intuitive." I had never heard those words before although they were soon to shape my destiny.

Since my fiancé had been killed, my life, I felt, was blown apart. To provide hope for my future, friends arranged a reading for me with an internationally renowned intuitive. During that reading she told me that I was going to "channel information," I had no idea what that meant. She also relayed that I would be able to see inside of human body like Superman's x-ray vision. Right!

A few days later I told a friend about the intuitive "reading." He said "OK, then look at my heart." So I said out loud, "I ask to see his heart." The next thing I knew, there all bright red and shiny superimposed over his body was his pumping heart with all the moving valves and his entire coursing vascular system. I turned pale white, and got so sick at my stomach that I had to sit down on the ground to avoid passing out! What was happening to me!?????????????????

I hid out in my room for several days afraid to deal with any more visuals like that again. Then I remembered the inituitive's predictions and decided to learn what she meant by "channel" and "see inside" bodies. I began my quest to LEARN what I was doing. And more importantly how to control it!

It took many years, multiple techniques, testings, and ongoing personal mental control and verbal command tools to learn how to harness, understand, direct and guide this magnificent Gift for the benefit of others. Otherwise this awesome ability called a "Gift" by some, a power by others and just plain weird by even more, would use me up and dominate my life.

In my seminars, workshops, webinars, seminars et al, I describe it like this: My Gift is a beautiful wonderful amazing wild stallion that is incredibly powerful. Either you learn how to ride and harness the stallion at YOUR direction, and know when to put him in the stable and lead a normal life, or that stallion will dominate and exhaust you and your life.

The following is the order of lessons I learned from the Universe and other teachers and educational materials, mostly the Universe. The Universe provided me with a Gift that activated when I wanted to "just do it!" I needed no training or certifications other than listening to Guidance. This was some incredible stuff to deal with!

I found that the Gift isolated me, yet gave me a higher connection and I learned 99% of all I know from asking the "voices in my head" to "show me" and provide the answers that I require in or to be accountable to, responsible for and the channel/ conduit of my humbling Gift.

I hope that you enjoy reading about my journey. I have tried to write it as if you are sitting in my presence having a conversation. My way of teaching is storytelling. All I know is what I've experienced. I hope my journey provides insight, clarity and assistance for your path.

I have found that all of my book's ideas and concepts about living with a Gift of intuitive healing energy and medical intuition boil down to a simple theory and assignment:

GO with who you are, BE who you are.
Don't let the lack of anything or knowledge or anyone tell YOU about what
YOU KNOW!
If you are truly a conduit,
JUST BE ONE!!
The Universe and God will do the rest!

Everything that you ever need to learn, see or know resides inside of you.

Your assignment is to:
1. Choose, accept, trust, protect, cleanse and allow the Gift to flow through you.

2. Show up with accountability, responsibility and integrity.

3. Follow the directives of your Higher Power and Guides and trust the information given to you.

4. Detach remove and release from your client and session. Go onto your next experience unfettered and unaffected by energy, issues or entities.

5. Go home and enjoy your life on earth!

Everything
you ever need
to learn, see or know,
resides
inside of you!

A "Gift"

So you think that you may have a "Gift." Or were born acknowledging that you had special talents, or everyone tells you that you are "gifted," or your life provided a sudden upheaval that awakened talents within you that had been simmering or were previously latent. Now your soul's yearning is creating a new life direction for you or amplifying what you have been doing with stealth like insurmountable persistence that you can't shake!

A Gift can also be initiated with inexplicable and sudden redirection of your life through an event. Sometimes when you are a success in your job or career, you "get" a medical situation, debilitating occurrence, or an unexpected sabbatical or job loss or something that changes and rearranges everything and everyone in your life.

During that experience, you begin to be drawn to a spiritual task and you have the emergence of new Gifts. It's the Universe directing your path to your soul's contract.

Since a Gift can wreak havoc with all areas of your being, I'm going to try to break it down to the areas that most folks ask questions about in all my forms of presentations. We're going to discuss the various things that you'll probably be addressing in your mind, emotions and life.

Always remember that your Gift will never be static unless you just shut down. Even **then**, the Universe or your Higher Power will be working in unforeseen ways. Gifts always evolve.

You may begin on one path and end up on many different avenues throughout your life.

Don't get so locked into a specific direction that you miss guidance that is reconfiguring even greater possibilities. Remember you are a spiritual being in a human body located on the human earth school. Your entire life process is your soul's journey and the choices you make will assist in configuring that adventure.

Let's start with the mental aspects. You have free will choice. You have a CHOICE to use your Gift in this incarnation. You can accept or reject your Gifts by free will choice and or set some or all of them aside for another embodiment. However if you have agreed to be a _____, then you have a contractual soul obligation with the Universe /Higher Power to fulfill.

Don't be a healer, intuitive, animal communicator, or whatever your Gift may embody because a reading "told you so." Don't use your Gift because your ego wants to do so. (Then the Gift is already "tainted," more about that later) Open to your soul's contract because it is your heart's desire and your soul's knowing.

If you grew up as a child with your Gift, you are in what they call the Contract A group, using your special talents early in life. Those of us that had Gifts activated later in life are the contract B activation group according to www.Lightworker.com archives.

Why would you not accept your Gifts? You are not required to use all of your Gifts. Use only those Gifts that resonate and create happiness while you use them. Just because you have lots of clothes in a closet, you don't have to wear them all at once. Neither do you have to experience and use all your Gifts at once.

A prayer for the Gifts you want to keep or shut down.
Since you are in charge of your body and Gifts, choose the specific Gift that you are addressing and the timeframe in which you want to use it, or not. You get to set the parameters of your Gifts involvement in your life.
State: Thank you for the Gift of _____. I do not choose to use _____ (name the Gift) at _____ (this time or choose a time frame, or in this incarnation) unless it for my highest and best good and protection. So be it. It is done! Thank you.

Let's presume that you have decided to use your Gift, How do you know what you'll be doing with it? Usually the random details and interests that you have been drawn to throughout your life are your calling. Additionally every bit of "training" that you have experienced up to this point will fuel the direction or focus of what you'd do. Example, if you were a drug addict, or always liked animals, or were drawn to flowers, usually all these cumulative experiences will provide the training for your client base that you will be working with.

Usually you'll work in the setting with the type of individuals that you have been around all your life. Your background in society, career, karmic path, environmental conditions, and previous issues that you have dealt with are all preparation for your work with the exact caliber of individuals who have issues that you have experienced. Your personal tests, testimonials and experiences have trained you for your specific clientele.

The affluent country club person usually has contacts in that group because they can relate to one another's lifestyle. A recovered alcoholic usually is the best AA mentor. An accountant may start their journey by initially helping office coworkers on the side until their career in healing assumes full blossom and requires they quit their "day job."

The Universe has spent a great deal of time educating you for your purpose, so what you've done is a large contributing factor to who, where, when and what type of client base will benefit from your service.

What you considered a hardship, dysfunctional; being "bad" was Universe training class 101. Everything that was horrific was graduate school exams! Everything that you ever experienced was the University of the Universe getting you ready to graduate into what you do with your Gift!

There will come a time when everything that you have ever done or participated in life will make sense and "jell." If you were a "wild" girl, and now have a calling, you'll probably be working with women who are in the same situation that you were involved in and have grown through. After I healed my fractured vertebrae and spinal issues I was swamped with spinal cord injury clients. So review your past history of learning; the good, bad and ugly. That information will usually provide the clearest directive of the service path most appropriate for you.

On the other hand, you may be jump starting a brand new direction, with only your soul's guidance prevailing in the winds of change. **The following prayer will help focus your path.**
State: I ask and it is my intent to bring in all people who will benefit from my Gifts and service to others, and to close the doors and remove all people that do not accelerate my path for my highest and best good. Please read this twice:

**No client base is more important than another;
it's just your directive for this incarnation.**

The individuals serving kings and queens, those serving the homeless, those working for free and the highly paid are all equal in the Universe's eyes. Each just has a different territory, assignment and pay scale for the relative client base served. Your Gift is unique to you and your service. If we all were the same then humanity's needs would have to be the same. Gifts come in various strengths and flavors to meet multiple needs.

The Emotional Side of the Gift

You've made the mental decision that you are going to accept your calling in this incarnation or a portion thereof.

Now doubt sets in. Why do I feel so alone? I really feel isolated and different when I'm supposed to be so loving and in service to others. Am I good enough, am I worthy? I'm afraid I might misuse my Gift. Ok, If I accept this Gift, is this real and what do I do with It, and there has to be downsides!

These are THE questions that plague most "newbies" including me!

So I had to figure out a way to get around or think through these emotional hurdles to my being in full service without reservations.

Personal Isolation: You are not alone in spirit, your energy has just shifted and you will be reconnecting under a different frequency. You feel detached, because you are not "feeling" your world and friends and others in the same familiar energy resonance pattern.

Gifted people usually learn to stand in their own power and to stand emotionally alone in order to trust their own intuition. Often they have come from a dysfunctional family, friends, and environmental background or other surroundings that create and require them to trust their own gut reactions.

Think about it, if there was a world catastrophe and you listened to everything and everyone's opinion, how could you make a great decision on how best to serve? On the other hand if you listened to your Higher Power and your guidance, the solution would be truly Divine and unaffected and unafflicted by circumstances.

When my Goddaughter was born with status epileptic seizures, at one point I was called to stabilize her heart rate and breathing while she awaited a Life Flight. When I went into the room there was a tiny fragile human being with more wires and monitors on her than there was body weight. I was so taken about, that I had to leave the room due to nausea and to keep my knees from collapsing from being so overcome with distraught grief and concern.

I was absolutely NO help to her as my human side engulfed my Gift.

Right then and there I decided I was going to "shake off" my human feelings and go in there and do what I came to do on Earth and to listen to my guidance.

I took a deep breath, and marched myself back into the room while saying my prayers. I worked fervently for the next 15 minutes until I had her heartbeat stabilized and her pulmonary function restored to a normal range where it stayed as the Life Flight loaded her aboard.

Then I went outside and had my human crying spell over what just happened. I learned the effectiveness of my Gift was diminished by getting caught up in personal feelings, other's circumstances and situations.

It's not that you can't care about what is going on, but you MUST remove yourself from having any expectations. (Which will taint the outcome or interpretations). You must learn to differentiate and discern that isolative and independent energy state that is the fullness of the Gift that you get to direct and deploy as a good thing. In time you will learn to embrace the very solitary and isolative cocoon that heralded the onset of a world with new and wonderful service opportunities. That "cocoon" is standing in your full power as a person and conduit.

Self worth: "I'm not worthy." It doesn't matter!
You got picked by God, the Universe or your Higher Power!
So you are the "Pickee."

Let's think this concept through in segments for clarity.
Who are you to question God's/ the Universe's/ Your Higher Power's judgment about picking you since "They" are omnipotent, all knowing et al. When you doubt, you're being conceited by basically telling God that He has poor judgment, made a mistake and chose the incorrect person when He picked you.

Are YOU so omnipotent that YOU can tell GOD that He was wrong in choosing you? God feels you are worthy.
That's ALL you need to KNOW!

It doesn't matter WHY you are the "Pickee." You are! That's all you need to understand and accept. Your designation is not going away in this incarnation if you choose to use your Gift!

If you do NOT choose to use your Gift in this life, you are still the "Pickee" until you have fulfilled that "Pickee" contractual agreement with the Universe/ Higher Power in an incarnation.

I suggest you quit trying to fight being the "Pickee." No matter what YOU think or feel, and since you ARE the "Pickee," decide this is the embodiment to shine!

I'm afraid I might misuse my Gift. Even though you've sorta accepted being the "Pickee," you now have fear of the responsibility of the Gift and its unknowns.

Have you ever thought that this might be the incarnation where you are the good guy and get to enjoy, be recognized for and celebrate what you have, rather than be burned, stoned or killed for those special talents?

An old sage told me not to feel afraid. I asked "why?" She stated that whatever we feared was what we had <u>already experienced </u>in another life, which was <u>why,</u> is was such a strong feeling in this lifetime. WE know from a past life what the down side was.

SO in **this** lifetime, because we had ALREADY, key word, already been through the bad with our Gift, we do not have to experience that learning opportunity from our Gift again. Whew!

This time, we get to enjoy our Gift and use it productively as we are directed.   This explanation made sense to and resonated with me. That logic quieted my mind on the "afraid I will do harm with my Gift" issue.

If you truly believe that each incarnation is the opportunity to learn and experience and have soul's growth for the next embodiment, then her valuable information will relieve your inner angst also.

Now let's look at how to use your Gift in full Trust, not just halfway believing that this is all true and really happening. If you are still in a stall pattern or represent yourself to be a Light worker but are not really honoring yourself and your Gifts by having internal self doubt and lack of complete trust, you're diluting your purpose.

Look at your age. Determine what percentage of your life you have already "used up" 45%, 60 %?? This will be a reality check.   So what are you going to do with the rest of your life and your Gift?

I suggest that since you have had a physical birthday for your body that you choose a date and commit to your **soul's birthday.** Celebrate each year like you do your physical birthday. Invite your friends to celebrate. Make an announcement and create a support system for you. On your soul's birthday make a promise to the Universe / God and commit to and state out loud:
"I will never process half beliefs and "sorta Trust" any more. I choose to progress and BE all I am and can be. I Live I AM, I TRUST!"

Halfway believing is like being half pregnant or saying I totally Trust what's happening in my life **except** when I fly in airplanes.

You have to give up worry 100%, and Trust 100% or you're diluting all that is available to you.

I suggest that you can also state to God/ the Universe /your Higher Power this declaration, affirmation and promise:
"I will no longer misrepresent myself to myself and others.
I choose to live and BE my soul's contract. I choose to trust and never go back to a lack of faith and self doubt from this moment forward. So be it, it is done!"

You'll be tested, count on it!
State to the test: "I've had my soul's birthday, and I TRUST, now, forever more and always!" Plus I don't have the courage to go back on my word to God!

Don't ever regress to doubt, commit to trust! If God/ the Universe / your Higher Power doesn't want you to do something they will either stop you, or provide enough free will choice failures that you will "get" that you are choosing the wrong pattern of actions.

From this point on, you are progressing on your path rather than just processing learning techniques and self doubt issues.

Again, when you don't' Trust 100%, you are diluting your "Pickee" abilities!

The stage is now set. You're determining the Gifts you want to use, and you accept that you choose to use your Gift in this incarnation in full Trust. **Now we need to determine how fast you want to "get on" with your new journey.**
Your heart wants to help and you're frustrated by not doing what you feel you came here to do since you've accepted your "assignment." You feel like you are "wasting your life." "All my Gifts have not come together. I feel like I have spent my entire life struggling and I don't know what I am doing." "I feel rejected by the Universe with all my Gifts that do not take off or get the positive feedback and support that I need to move forward."
You get to direct your life forward UNLESS the Universe wants you to do this RIGHT NOW full on! I know a lady that was stuck in Canada with a car that needed to be repaired for her journey. She took a waitress job to add extra income. One day she was talking with a customer who asked if she believed in fortune telling and she said

yes. The customer said "why don't you just tell me what you see in my future?" not expecting any results.

Information erupted out of her! The customer sat stunned at the accuracy of detail and knowledge about her life.
The customer then went home and told another friend. Within a week, this woman was giving 25 readings a day for free and was so tired she had to quit waitressing. Almost broke, she started charging for her readings and the rest of the story- she is a renowned international intuitive. The Universe wanted her in service RIGHT NOW!!! If that is the case with you, "They" will provide absolutely everything that you need to do what "They" want you to do.

If you're not "on demand," your next choice is to monitor the speed of your progression into service or to accelerate it. First, you need to honor your path. If you don't honor you path, why should anyone else?

State: Send all those people and experiences to me now that will amplify my soul's contract and open all doors for my highest and best good. Remove any and all people, pledges, experiences, promises or past life commitments that hinder my path, now forevermore and always. So be it, it is done! Thank you!

Second, is there is anything holding you back?
When you get to the point of what you think is "failing" or not fast enough ask for Trust and to find or be shown another way to go forward. Do not fold your tent; ask to be shown another way.

This is also "Their" way of teaching you to ask for directives, information and guidance and to learn that you'll get quicker results by going straight to the source!

Prayer for your soul's path.
State: Dear God, close any and all doors, stop any and all activities, remove any and all energies and entities now and in all of time and all there is, that are not for my highest and best good and that are interfering and impeding my soul's path. Direct me now on my soul's path.

This cuts the Karmic timing and processing, and starts you actual progressing path. Be all you are and can be, not one iota less!!!!! Shine, shine, shine!

Third, remember since you are in the physical body you can always ask for acceleration or slowing down during your Soul's Path. Be careful and ready for the unexpected when you ask for that acceleration. Ask and be very specific about the type of acceleration that you want.

State: I ask and it is my intent for the Universe to accelerate my path now or _____ now. So be it, it is done.

I tested this theory one day while walking my dog. I asked for an acceleration of clients, the next day I had 23 + calls. Most of my sessions require 5 or more hours, which is different from an hourly appointment practice. So a few days later I chose to request that "They" hold off new clients for a while. They did! Then I told Them, "I'm ready to go back to work." And that's how I regulate the speed of my business unless I'm given a Higher Objective and specific timeframe assignment. I just Trust that everything will work out and I'll get to rest at the appropriate time!

Of note: Once you establish a work and life path flow pattern, don't be overly concerned during a lull or a pause in your path. The Universe is lining up all the myriad details within your journey. During the slow times you have an opportunity to do humanly chores, those domestic errands and catch up on personal details and human life activities. Then be prepared for more progressing on your path. KNOW that after the lull, almost always the fast, full pace resumes.

Attitude: Gift versus Ego/ Power

Some people allude to having "powers." "Power" is ego thinking and taints the very energy that you channel. A lot of individuals claim their Gift to be a power not realizing they have just diminished their wattage by adding a filter of ego over their previously clear avenue for being a conduit. I suggest that you be the steward of your "Gift" that channels thru you and not use your "Gift" as your ego empowerment

The next phase after all that decision making and choosing directives for your life is about responsibilities to be the best you can be!

Part 1

As the "Pickee" your job is:
To choose, accept, trust, protect,
cleanse and allow
the Gift
to flow through you.

Responsibilities for the Life You Have Chosen

Your primary responsibility is divided into three categories of taking care of the leased body your soul resides in and through which your Gift flows. They are Protecting/ Shielding, Cleansing and Allowing.

Protecting yourself as needed in my opinion, requires getting your prayers and intent on a specific tract. Let's look at how to pray in order to carefully craft and direct our prayers.

How to Pray: Be SPECIFIC!

The Universe lives in forever time and your leased vehicle (body) lives in finite time, so you need to be very specific. State:

I ASK: "ask and ye shall receive." It's a Universal Law that all those in charge of your soul's contract must respond. You're asking all those in charge of your soul to help you, now! Why not use ALL the powers you have on heaven and earth that are available to you???

It is MY INTENT (with a "T" NOT Intend) that brings your prayers into the NOW, in this incarnation, at this very moment in time. YOU MUST BE SPECIFIC!!!!!!!!!!!!!!!!
They live in forever time and in all that is, so be VERY specific about exactly what you want and in the VERY SPECIFIC timeframe of what you want. Not being specific (intend) is never never land, or "which incarnation?" etc. to those on the other side.

I suggest that you say your prayer 3 times. 3 is the universal number. The first time it set your free will to ask for help, the second time your prayer creates intent and the third time to me, means you're really focused on getting this done.

Use the words Now, Forevermore and Always.

"Now," brings your prayer into the now, i.e. present. The Universe operates in a timeless forever and to have Them respond to your command you must state "now", otherwise your guides will be asking "in which incarnation do you want this done?"

"Forevermore," takes the prayer into all energy realms, incarnations, and time frames.

"Always," makes the prayer results continuous with no time lapses.

At the finale of your request state: So be it, it is done.

Thank you. "So be it," brings the prayer into the present life situation. "It is done," manifests that the prayer has become and IS a reality, NOW!

If you are asking for a confirmation, or to be shown something, ASK for a specific time and for a specific number of confirmations within that timeframe. I suggest 3 confirmation signs within 24, 48 or 78 hours. Be sure to ask that these confirmations are shown to you in a manner that you as a human can understand as your confirmation. What God may feel is really obvious, you at this point, may not understand. Ask that you be able to see, recognize, and understand the confirmation.

If you do NOT get any confirmations, then KNOW that it may not be the time for you to have and answer, or try again and ask another way...........

When your prayers are answered, you have the support of formidable crowd with the Universe and "all there is." If you feel that you ask and pray for answers too much, remember, there is a place in the Universe where your unasked questions are, the Gifts that you never requested and the guides you never used. Use all there is that is available to you and your soul's contract. ASK!

Armed with the knowledge of how to construct prayers for maximum results, the first thing to do every day, is to protect the body that your soul resides in.

Protecting/ Shielding: Think of it this way: your soul is a bright and shining light like the light in a lighthouse. Your body surrounds and houses your soul, like the lighthouse encompasses its light. Your soul shines out of your eyes like the light shines out of the lighthouse glass.

Your soul is protected, because you are a part of all that is. However, your body is not protected from the experiences of the earth school, like the lighthouse is not protected from its environment. Therefore you have to protect your soul's housing like the light keeper protects and maintains his lighthouse.

Your energy's residence can be shielded in a bubble/ cocoon of protective energy created through your intent. Think of the clear glass around a "snow ball." Its contents on the inside are totally enveloped in that cocoon no matter what else is happening around the world outside of that glass parameter. As your "Light keeper," within this bubble/ cocoon you are protected as you control life and direct your actions.

Cocooning yourself in this protective bubble puts you in full control and charge of all that is available to you. When you are in your director's room enclosure, you are standing in full empowerment.

Being in this bubble YOU control your energy's flow. YOU allow what affects you into your life. Like Bob Barker, you can open the door and say "come on down" to bad energy and negative energies or entities. Or you can only open and allow your director's room to be made available to people, events and environments that are for your highest and best good!

NO energy or entity can ever affect you unless you allow it. You might want to paste that on your refrigerator! Memorize it in your being. Plus, this saves an ENORMOUS amount of energy in defending yourself and warding off detrimental energies or entities! You can use that extra energy that would have been expended on negative energies to use for enjoying life or amping up your Gifts.

State: I ask and it is my intent, to surround myself in a seamless mirrored--(bubble or cocoon) of the Christ White Light (or whomever is your Higher Power), to protect me now, forevermore, and always, and to only allow the energy or entities which is for my soul's highest and best good to come thru. So be it, it is done. Thank you.

Why do I use the word seamless? Seamless means nothing comes in or out unless you allow it. The concept of mirrored means that any negative energy or entity, event or whatever that is aimed at you, reflects back to the sender so that you will not be drained or affected. SO easy!

Who and what can be shielded is everything, anything and anyone. The protection bubble can be placed around you, your house, brother, pet, car, airplane, your travel's path et al, hotel room, and even another person (to use as they choose to use so you do not interfere with their free will choice).

If you need an extra protection boost or a quickie shield use this method. With or without verbiage with your sending palm facing outwards, start at your root charka and make a rainbow arc that goes up to and over your head while, setting your intent to and say " shield, shield, shield." I use this while saying "hi" to negative persons, or while standing in front of the microwave heating my tea.

I suggest that you always maintain an awareness of integrating your energy field with everything around you. If you feel "off" or an unspecified thing is affecting you, you have allowed something to affect your control room!

Shield immediately then clean them out (see later in the chapter). **You** choose your awareness level which creates or depletes your energy and empowerment.

Being slack on protection and cleansing will create an energy drain and build up that will make you tired. It will allow your energy to be siphoned and will impair your ability to be a conduit. I surround myself every morning and extra in hospitals or draining environments or people. Folks ask "why do you spend so much time with this shielding?"

My answer is twofold. First, it takes less time than brushing your teeth, and you can say it while brushing your teeth. Secondly to have the full embodiment of my Gift at all times is to me, hardly an exchange for protecting its residence.

It's your choice on how often you take care of or neglect protecting your "all you can be!" I have myriad clients who come for me to work with them because they have "burned out," "stay tired all the time" or aren't "progressing and moving forward."

The first thing I ask is do they shield and protect their Gift. They usually say, "My soul is protected, so why bother." And if they do some sort of protective ritual you can bet their verbiage is "never never land" non specific for any guides to complete in this incarnation. Then I ask do your protect the body your soul resides in, and they say "why?" or "oh I don't do that."

The difference between long term extraordinary and ordinary is the way you take care of and maintain the protection of your Gift!

Shielding Yourself against Other Things

Emergency situations always present chaotic energy. I always add an extra layer of shielding while working under that form of duress. To be safe while activating your healing energy as quickly as possible **state**:

Surround me, shield me, fill me, and ground me to do your work now. Use me, use me, use me.

This will immediately connect you to your guidance and activate your energy when there is no time for meditation, warm up techniques, et al.

Medical and healthcare facilities retain all the energy that ever was in, on and around their grounds and buildings. Think about that! Shield yourself before you enter any healthcare facility. Clear the room you are working in and fill it with positive and physically healing and healing energy. You can even put the room, hospital and client in a bubble if your client is going to remain in that location.

You can shield an operating room to control the energy of that area including each physician, nurse and other staff. But you must state that the bubbles' protection is to be used "as they so choose and only for their highest and best good." In that manner you are not interfering with any Karma. All rooms hold all of the energy and entities that were ever in that room.

While leaving healthcare facilitates I suggest clearing, releasing and detaching any and all energies and entities from your energy field as you walk to your next destination.

"Energy vampires" are always there. Dark is always there because it balances Light. Both have to cohabit for the other to exist. Everything is energy. If you don't shield, everything that needs energy will try to siphon your life force energy.

I call dark energy "Moths" because they are attracted to light. As an example: when you turn on your back porch light at night, think of how many moths come to that light. When you go to a stadium game, think about the thousands of moths attracted to the greater wattage lights. Whew!

"Moths" create balance. The greater your Light, the more the "moths" for balance. For those of you who have experienced entity and energy "blobs" at night, protect yourself by

1. Asking who they are (it's a Universal law that they must answer)
2. Ask who they serve.
3. Then command them away by saying:

State: I ask and it is my intent and I command you to leave my space now forevermore and always. So be it, it is done.

The Universe is set up that all energies and entities (living or deceased) are required to respond to the free will choices for your space. To remove anything that you do not want in or occupying your space use the prayer above. I suggest 3 times!

FYI

An easy way to have continuous protection that has been used since time began is a sterling silver cross. As an illustration, Monks wore a cross at their groin (root chakra) and nuns wore them over their heart area. Sterling silver repels negative energy. I wear a sterling silver cross over my heart area. It removes all things negative, but MUST have a plain clean undecorated surface on the silver so negative energy can be mirrored back to the sender.

Cleansing Your Body & Surroundings

Physically, your body bumps into the energies of EVERYTHING and entities as you move throughout life like those waves and salt spray in the Lighthouse scenario. Every person that you have interfaced with in your life has created an impression and an ongoing connection in your energy field unless you remove them. Every client you have even come into contact with is plugged into in your energy field until you release and detach from them.

Think about that concept. If you are a conduit and your pipeline is overlaid with multiple veils of energy and entities, you are being drained by a gazillion active connections. And you wonder why you are tired and channel less energy? Imagine your conduit ability IF you were like a clean PVC pipe with water flowing through it.

Or is your pipeline one that has hundreds of screens over the initial portal with sludge throughout the pipe, mold on the walls and septic residue at the end. Now you want to channel energy to of for a client consultation and wonder WHY "it's not as effective as it used to be."

Clean your bubble shield every night perhaps while cleaning your teeth or just before you fall asleep. It's like cleaning a windshield of the car that has bugs embedded in the windshield grime that accumulated throughout your day.

The most effective routine, I find, to maintain the highest quality and quantity of ongoing energy and channeling excellence is to shield every morning, and detach, remove and release energy and entities each night. Practicing this will give you more energy.

If you're lazy with this maintenance routine, just remember, the brighter Light you are, the more "moths" you attract that can erode "all you are and can be," and you'll be covered in client sludge.

This is a quickie prayer to clean your energy field.
State: I ask and it is my intent to remove, release and detach any and all energies and entities from my energy field now, forevermore and always and to send them to the Christ White Light (or your Higher Power). So be it, it is done.

Your energy field bubble needs to be cleaned just from "living your life" debris from time to time. Make an appointment with yourself to clean your energy field on a regular basis of at least once a month.

Another method to physically clean your energy field.

Put 1/4 cup of sea salt or Epsom salt, (unless you have known sensitivities to either) in your bath water, and stay in that water for ONLY 15 minutes. Staying in the water longer will deplete your energy. This helps remove toxins from your energy field.

If this is not possible, just take a short shower and let the water cleanse your field or you can hand spray yourself (like a Windex bottle) with salt water while showering.

Set your intent and state to yourself that the water is removing and releasing and detaching all energy and entities et al...

My advice to energy workers:
1. Remove, release and detach your clients on an appointment by appointment and daily basis. You can do this by running water over your wrists for a few minutes between client sessions.
2. Remove daily debris with your cleansing prayer
3. Physically clean your full energy field at least once a month.

Another prayer to remove energy from your energy field or your house, furniture, land, property et al.
State: I ask and it is my intent and I command the energy to remove, release and detach any and all excess, unnecessary, preexisting, toxic or unhealthy energy or entities from _____ now forevermore and always. I ask the energy be replaced with the healing loving energy of the Christ white light (or whomever is your power source), now, forevermore and always. So be it, it is done. Thank you.

48

Allowing- Ready to Work

You've accepted your assignment and now have a client, that's when the self doubt sets in. Set your intent to "Use me" and ask to allow the energy of your Gift whatever that may be, to flow thru you.

God doesn't care how you heal or how you communicate. He just wants you to do what resonates with your free will choice under His guidance. Your training and Gift job description is specified for the exact clientele that you are sent.

There is no competition. No work is insignificant.

No one can diminish your Gifts. Only <u>you</u> can create the doubt that impedes the Universal flow thru you. Ask to fine tune your Gifts. If you like your direction and it feels correct, push forward in that direction. The Universe will redirect you with free will choice "nudgies," if you are not on course.

My specialty in distant energy healing appears to be electromagnetic. When I started working with nerve regeneration and restoral of nerve function, I loved it! Stopping seizures half a world away was gratifying. Then I moved on to channeling the energy which reversed paralysis. That was so incredibly humbling to look into a client's face filled with disbelief and see them very childlike and gleefully practice the function that was once lost now restored.

My first client, a mother of 2 teenage boys, was told she would never walk again due to progression from MS to Devic's Disease. After about 20 minutes, she could move her legs. I will never forget the look on her face. I went home and stared at my hands for several days, afraid to touch anything. That's when I knew it was NOT me, and my Gift was serious!

To this day, I feel so privileged and blessed to be a conduit for this work. However I can't fix bladder infections (unless it's an electromagnetic stimulation issue).

Everything has its place and the order of go in which the Universe wants your Gift to benefit others.

Later on my path I received more and more clients that wanted a medical intuitive body scan. When I was looking into bodies, after getting over the initial ugly graphics of it, I knew I had found my calling, I loved it, I was humbled by it, I loved it and I love it!!!!!

You'll know when you have arrived at where you belong. And then it's possible you'll be egged into another direction like I'm writing this book to help activate your Gifts, and educate you in ways to further your career.

I never thought I would be doing this, until I realized that I had minored in Creative Writing! No coincidence there............the Universe was training me 40 years ago for now!

Always know that when you allow the Universe to work through you,

**if you heal or affect even only one person in your life
for their highest and best good, you have done a great job.**

It's not necessary to completely cease and desist what you are currently doing, just because you have a calling for your Gift. You can maintain your current career and contribute to friends, colleagues and strangers. Consider that you may have come to earth for both callings. You can also be highly and terrifically Gifted and only use it once. Your agreement with the Universe determines your course in this incarnation.

Although this book is about intuitive healing and medical intuition, Gifts come in all flavors: laughter, hiring people, art, philanthropic interests, saving the earth or animals and a simple pat on the back "atta boy/girl" to someone who needed your comment at that precise moment in time!

Allow what you and the Universe have agreed upon and don't feel "less than" ever!

Part 2

Show up
with
accountability, responsibility,
and
integrity.

(State this at top of the page)
Client Release and Contract   Page 1 of 2
Client Release and Contract   on   date
Please fill required spaces marked with the red X
between
Your Name and

X _____("Client") of
        Please print Name

X _____Full Address

I understand that Your Name of your business is an type of business and does not present herself as a medical doctor nor as possessing any formal medical training, nor as a licensed, registered or certified practitioner or counselor. (Leave out some verbiage if you are certified)

In consideration of the promises and conditions contained herein, I seek and it is my intent to hire Your Name for what you do. As further consideration for Your Name's Services, I agree to provide certain current, complete and accurate information about myself as required on Your Name's client information form. No one representing your business or Your Name offers me any false hope, false promises, expectations, warranties, or assurances of the success or the outcome of any of Your Name's work.

I have read and understand Your Name fees and that they are pre paid BEFORE my appointment is scheduled, and non refundable. I agree to the payment conditions and to pay the total fee amounts for Your Name's services in US Funds.

I choose the following service (s). Please write clearly
    1. _____   Fee: _____ X

    2. _____   Fee:_____
Additional Fees if applicable: Emergency : _____
                            Travel:_____

Initial Total fees are: _____ X
If I pay by debit or credit card , I understand that by providing the following information to YOUR NAME and YOUR COMPANY that I agree to and I legally authorize that the debit or credit card below be charged to pay for Your Name's Consultation(s), answers to Email questions and or Energy Medicine.

If I pay via PayPal, I agree to and authorized that transaction to pay for YOUR NAME services.

The PayPal email address is YOUR EMAIL ADDRESS

I understand and agree to the following: a. if I need to reschedule my appointment, that I am required to give Ms Atwater's office a 24 hour notice. b. If I miss my appointment, without giving Your Name's office a 24 hour notice for rescheduling, I will be charged the full fee for your business activities and_or Travel arrangements. c. I phone Your Name for my sessions and pay the charges.

I am eighteen (18) years of age or older, of sound mind, and not under any mind altering drugs. By signing this agreement, I acknowledge that I have read the above, have thoroughly reviewed and   understand its contents, and that I am giving my informed consent and it is my intent to agree to this   contract. By my written acceptance of this agreement, I know this document becomes a legally binding contract and is confidential. This Contract shall be governed by and construed in accordance with the laws of the State of YOUR STATE.

X Signature: _____ Seal
    Date: _____ X
    Witness: _____

Consent by Legal guardian, Parent or Attorney in Fact.

As the Parent and or Legal Guardian, or POA, I acknowledge that I have read the above, have thoroughly reviewed and understand its contents, and that I am giving my informed consent. It is my intent to agree to this contract.   I authorize you to provide services for:
_____ (Client).

X Signature: _____ Seal
    Date: _____

X Witness: _____

Your Company Logo and Name
Address
Town, State, Zip code
Office Phone: Fax:
Email:

Client Release and Contract on   date   page: 2 of 2
Be sure to fill in the required spaces marked with the red X

My payment method for my appointment(s) is: Please check one of the
following
Personal Check:_____ Money Order:____ Pay Pal:_____
Credit or Debit Card:_____ Type of card:_____

     X Name as it appears on the card:_____

     X Card number, Please Print CLEARLY:_____

     X Expiration date of card :_____

     X The last three numbers on signature strip:_____

The Billing Name and Address as it appears on the card's statements:
  X _____
  X _____
  X _____
  X _____

You will receive instructions for your appointment(s) when it is
scheduled. Thank you.

Disclaimer:
Disclaimer: YOUR NAME is not a medical doctor nor associated with
any branch of allopathic medicine. YOUR NAME is a DESCRIPTION OF
YOUR WORK. YOUR NAME DESCRIPTION OF YOUR WORK opinions are
based on HIS/HER intuition and should not be a substitute for a
medical examination and are not a substitute for medical procedures
or treatments.
ALWAYS consult a physician or trained health care professional
concerning diagnosis for any medical problem or condition and before
undertaking any diet, health related or lifestyle change programs.
As in traditional medicine, there are no guarantees with YOUR WORK.

Business name, address etc information as header

Client Information Form   All client information is strictly confidential and secure.   Please fill this out completely, and Mail, Fax or email to address listed above. Thank you

CLIENT NAME:_____ _____
(last name first)   first   nickname

PARENT'S NAME:_____

CLIENT BIRTH DATE:_____ TIME:_____
PLACE:_____

OCCUPATION:_____
Please include CLIENT PHOTO: _____

HOME ADDRESS:_____
_____
_____

HOME PHONE:_____ EMAIL HM: _____

HOME PHONE 2:_____ CELL:_____
OFFICE PHONE:_____ EMAIL OFF:_____

PET'S NAME:_____
SPECIES_____ AGE_____
 Your pet's Picture (if it's the client) :_____

Alternative contact:_____
Phone:_____

Referring Physician /Specialist/
Practitioner (s):_____ __

A good time to call to schedule your appointment _____
IS Email communication easy for you?_____
What are convenient times for your appointment?_____

May I use your or your pet's photos WITHOUT names on my website? _____

Time-Zone Converter link for your time zone appointments

Your Name- Client Information Form p 2

If you are having a Medical Intuitive Diagnostic Imaging session (Body Scan), please do not tell me your issues so I will have no preconceived ideas, images or opinions.

What issues do you want addressed?
This section is not necessary if _____

_____

_____
_____
_____

Who are your Medical / Holistic and Integrative providers?

_____
_____
_____
_____

What Alternative treatments are you currently working with?

_____
_____
_____

What Medicines or Herbs are you currently taking?

_____
_____ _____
_____

Additional Comments about things that you would like me to know that you feel would be helpful information.

Preparing Your Client for the Appointment

After the client has sent in their initial paperwork, I suggest you sent out a time schedule and confirmation letter providing the time or times that you have or can be available for them and include instructions for their forthcoming appointment.

Below is the Confirmation Letter form I send to my clients when I have processed their payment and secured a time slot on my calendar for them. You are welcome to use any sections that are appropriate for your business.

****

Business Heading
Full Address
Phone & Fax
Email

Thank you for choosing my work as part of your healthcare and healing journey. Your information has been received and your payment has secured your appointment.

Between receipt of your application and timing of your actual appointment getting scheduled on my calendar varies - sometimes a few days, 2-3 weeks, or other times it's longer.

** In order to guarantee your time slot, ASAP please confirm that you received your instructions and are able to comply with your appointment time. **

Although I appreciate and understand your enthusiasm in your healing journey, please do not call me to see when your appointment is scheduled. Please do not send multiple "nudgie" emails or call to see if I have received your emails.

I will address any questions that have arisen in our next session. All appointments are set at the appropriate time to facilitate your healing journey. If I need to change your appointment time I will notify you beforehand in ample time.

INITIAL INFORMATION:

1. Please don't forget to email or mail me your photo BEFORE our session.

Do NOT fax your photograph, as it appears only as a gray indiscernible "blob".

2. I ask that you give my office a 24-hour notice to reschedule your appointment. Otherwise you will be charged your full fee.

BEFORE APPOINTMENTS:

BEFORE your appointment, please check your phone messages and email.

** If I am called for an emergency, I will do my best to notify you.

PHONE at your appointment's Eastern Standard Time, the number I have provided.

Convert your Eastern Standard Time appointment time to YOUR local time zone.

International clients may want to use their late night free cell phone hours, a prepaid card or other calling card for low rates.

DELAYS: Sometimes my schedule gets backed up. Please allow a 30-minute leeway around your appointment time. If the phone is busy at our appointed time, wait a few minutes and try again. Do not call my mobile phone to see why my office phone is busy. I will answer as soon as possible.

Since I have a lot of clients on multiple medications, under duress and in medical situations that might affect their clarity, I provide the following Instructions for my clients. You might want to make a set of Instructions for your clients.

CONSULTATION & ENERGY HEALING:

1. We will have a consultation to identify your health issues.
2. We will mutually choose during our consultation a time when I will run the energy part of our session. I prefer to run the energy at night so your body will have more time to recalibrate.

BODY SCAN Medical Intuitive Diagnostic Imaging™:

At your appointment's designated Eastern Standard Time, please call the number provided: _____

Prior to your MIDI and or Energy Healing

I ask that you take a bath. Put 1/4 cup of sea salt or Epsom salt, (unless you have known sensitivities to either) in your bath water and stay in that water for ONLY 15 minutes or your energy will be depleted. This helps cleanse your energy field. If this is not possible, just take a short shower and set your intent to let the water cleanse your field.

1. I prefer for you to be in a QUIET environment, without any distractions, and that you not have anyone else near you during our session. You may have a pet in the room.

2. Please refrain from eating heavy or greasy food, and drinking alcohol or smoking 24 hours prior to our session.

3. Please refrain from eating 1 hour before I do Energy Work with you.

4. I would also prefer that you have not had another energy treatment at least 3 days prior to our session as your body may still be adjusting to the recalibration of the another treatment or procedure, or 5 days after due to your frequency recalibration. (Emergencies are an exception).

What to Expect:

You remain fully clothed, however I ask that you remove all watches, and anything metal that you might be wearing. I prefer that you are barefooted.

Have your palms facing upwards and do not cross your hands or feet. Crossing your hands or feet disrupts the Energy flow and releasing toxic unhealthy energy.

For personal safety, if you are having on site energy healing done, I ask that you allow 30 minutes to remain stationery after your energy work before you drive, or that you have someone with you who can drive you to your destination.

Energy healing at night:

I prefer to schedule your energy work while you sleep. During sleep your body recalibrates itself. If you have a sleeping partner, please ask them to be in another location/room for the first hour of your energy healing. This keeps the Energy focused on you, and not diluted by someone sharing your field. Please remove any bedside phones, remotes, or clocks on "your" side.

After your Energy work:
I ask that you drink water with lemon juice in it for 3 days following our session, unless you are intolerant to lemons or their chemical content, or have any other factors that would
prohibit their use (meds, or a disorder). This keeps your electrolytes balanced while your body is releasing, restoring & adjusting to your new frequencies.

Thank you.

That Place Between Allowing and Working

There is a place for a split second or longer when you have made all the choices, have chosen to Trust, yet that human self doubt about what you can and can't do eases its way into your mind.

"I'm not sure what I am doing." YES YOU ARE.

Your human ego "thinks you don't know what you are doing".

YOUR SOUL KNOWS exactly what you are doing! Ask for Guidance.

Self doubt, your ego, and self expectation issues create governors that diminish your "flow" and Gifts.

It's NOT your job to know "how to do it." God/ the Universe/ Your Higher Power know how to flow the energy and provide the information and instructions to get the job done in the exact manner with the EXACT appropriate outcome.

How do I determine if the "voices in my head" are guidance and not ego? Even though a modality may activate your Gifts, your inner knowing and intuition, your inner guidance will always lead you. Always listen to your heart and what resonates in your heart.

Guidance is a definite and different tone delivered in a soft yet firm directive manner. To insure that you are listening to your guidance **state:**

I ask and it is my intent to set aside my ego and open my heart in Trust so I can hear my guidance with complete unfiltered clarity. SO be it, it is done!

Ask who the voice(s) work for; the Light, the dark?

Guidance is required to answer. Sometimes if you have not shielded yourself and prepared correctly to allow the information to flow through you, you become a portal for energies and entities that have a freeway to come into the earth plane through you without reservation or boundaries and communicate as they choose. NOT good! I say a VERY specific prayer before every session to take care of this issue. You'll find it in a later chapter.

Oftentimes while you are allowing the flow of the Gift through you, you will know you are doing everything correctly and communicating appropriately by various means of **confirmations from the Universe**.

Chills, tingles, hair rising on your neck or other reoccurring signals that are individually yours mean confirmation from the Universe that what you are hearing or experiencing from Them or the client or the situation is "right on" solid Truth! Some people call goose bumps "God" bumps☺.

Before you work with your Gift you need to be aware of the downside of sensitivity. The downside of extra ordinary sensitivity is that you have a heart and a body that is empathetic and sympathetic, which makes you vulnerable.

Your "sensitivity" is what facilitates and substantiates your Gifts. Shielding yourself will prevent you taking on anyone else's, energy or problems and will still maintain your ability to read then and be empathetic towards the energy that you are reading. The most important part is that shielding will keep their energy mess out your energy field.

Many healers say, "I'm so tired after I have worked all day." Obviously they do not know how to shield themselves and orchestrate their energy correctly. A lot of intuitive energy healers like the "drama" of being affected by their work and being humanly depleted by their "powers" or their quintessential sensitivity.

My take is that they do not manage their Gift correctly and are degrading themselves. *It's not a badge of honor to be possessed by your Gift!*

The energy you are spending on drama or being effected could be spent on facilitating healing someone. Drama around energy work or healing is a waste of your energy. You don't get "points" for being so sensitive you are "affected", you only get "points" for doing your work to benefit others.

Sometimes your sensitive sonar system which is how you "feel" energy's vibrational frequency creates panic attacks, heart palpitations et al because your energy system's sensitivity is overloaded and unshielded. Shield!

These are fun exercises to practice maneuvering your energy field's sonar system.

Set your intent to pull your energy field in so you are indiscernible and have a friend try to locate you. Set your intent to "beam up" or locate a consenting friend. This little practice tool teaches you to "find" energy fields, which is how you learn to feel your client's vibrational frequency no matter where they are located. You can do this with your pets. Intuitive energy workers who locate lost individuals and pets or even corpses are pros at this technique!

Now it's time to show up and go to work!

The Different Medical Intuitive Body Scans

This book is about how medical intuition is used for diagnosis and how to see, locate, examine and discern the bioenergy patterns of diseases, disorders, medical conditions and health issues.

For those advanced individuals, bear with us. For those of you who are beginning to learn, I'm starting at the basics and building a foundation of understanding on how to use these tools and techniques and in my opinion, why you want to use them in the order I present them.

An intuitive medical body scan is generally accepted to be the use of your inner intuition and senses to gather information about your client's energy systems throughout their cellular blueprint. To me, you're scanning the scrapbook of the theater of their body's life.

There are several forms of medical intuitive scans. A medical intuitive scan can present a single perspective or a multi level evaluation since your energy field and bimolecular structures store all things that have happened to and will occur to you in this life and many that are from past incarnations.

This book's intuitive scans deal with this incarnation's energy. The difference to me between a medical intuitive reading, a medical intuitive body scan and medical intuitive diagnostic imaging™ (MIDI) is described below.

Intuitive Diagnosis and a medical intuitive health assessment reading is when the practitioner tunes into the client's energy field. He answers questions and gives opinions from the intuitive information he "receives." The practitioner does not actually look into the cells or at an organ et al. The practitioner also offers intuitive suggestions for the health issues.

An intuitive Body Scan reviews the client's energy field and physical systems by intuitively evaluating the generalized overall energy patterns and the "feel" of those energy patterns. The practitioner reports their intuitive overview, evaluates the client's condition and addresses emotional and health issue questions without going into minute detail by actually seeing the tissue, bones, nerves, et al. They perceive the overall bioenergy field and note imbalances within that field. This is a great method for a yearly check up because I can compare last year's impressions with the current ones. This is like a doctor taking general blood work, having annual tests and x-rays.

I pioneered and founded the field of **MIDI-Medical Intuitive Diagnostic Imaging™.** It's the process of how to see inside a body to interpret the physical bioenergy patterns that identify and diagnose the energy codes of past, current and future diseases and health issues. It takes "inner vision," the term coined by Barbara Brennan, to an advanced level of detailed images.

A MIDI begins with a general Body Scan that is used as a baseline to tune into the client's energy field. Then like a MRI, the intuitive examines each physical energy layer in a specific area slice by slice to identify and interpret what created or is creating the cumulative effect that becomes the physical disorder.

The MIDI process is a very precise head to toe, front to back, over and under, 360 degree look inside the body. By examining each energy layer in a specific area slice by slice, the practitioner can learn to identify and interpret what created or is creating the cumulative effect that becomes the physical disorder. A MIDI reading generates an incredibly detailed and accurate location, size, description and determines the medical urgency associated with each illuminated health issue, in addition to providing a comprehensive diagnostic evaluation along with a future prognosis. A MIDI consultation can also supply suggestions for ongoing health management, medications, treatments and procedures from its database.

I LOVE the Body's theater!!!!! I LOVE my work! It is thrilling, awesome and humbling!

There is no difference to me, whether the MIDI is performed onsite or remotely for a client who is in a different location. Some practitioners are better with their client's being in their presence in order to discern their frequencies and energy patterns. Sometimes to promote confidence, a client prefers to physically be in your energy field and watch you work. This usually helps them confirm their answers are being facilitated by you.

Other practitioners are as adept at local viewing as well as distance or remote viewing of their client's energy field. I prefer distant viewing because I am not distracted by the client's personal details which allow me to focus more intensely and intently on their health issues.

The Value of Medical Intuition

Medical intuition can provide information about treatment, procedures, and appropriate medication dosages for patient physical conditions, age levels and current body weight (especially prevalent in geriatric medicine and some extensive Cancer or other chronic or degenerative diseases and disorders regimes).

Medical intuition supports patient advocacy, second opinions and expands the patient's holistic evaluation.

• It SAVES TIME! in catastrophic or trauma injury, critical or intensive care or emergency medicine situations.

• It can be performed from a distant location.

• Clarifies physical health and emotional issues and identifies critical disease areas or other energy imbalances.

• Identifies disease locations, determines the extent and severity in your body's disorder from a 360 degree energy view.

• Determines the "urgency" of your physical situation.

• Can continuously monitor the client's condition on site or at a distance.

• Has no side effects and is non invasive.

• Can confirm medical test results.

• Can be used in conjunction or in comparison with your current MRIs, PETs, MUGAs, CT Scans and X rays, et al.

• Can identify areas that have not yet become detectable by traditional medical examinations or testing. This information can assist you in making decisions about your medical treatment, and health care.

• Can provide information about future health issues.

All medical intuitive assessments are an invaluable tool. By identifying the causes of your current symptoms one can possibly prevent future health events or keep health issues, disorders or conditions from manifesting into physical dis-ease.

When Can a MIDI be Used?

A body scan and MIDI can be performed at any time, under any circumstances, anywhere in the world from my location. You can be on the operating table, riding a bike, having wine in Paris, or being in the process of transition. The body's energy field is informative, steadfast and readable, in an around your physical body up to, through, and until you have completely transitioned into another energy form on the other side.

What Can Affect Client's Energy Information?

We have scientifically documented that energy is JUST as strong and available to be read remotely as on site if the intuitive has that frequency range ability. One can actually focus more quickly because you're not looking at the client's personal details and your surroundings. But some things do affect your reading.

Personal Blockages:

Did you know that RUBBER STOPS THE FLOW OF ENERGY!!!! Think about it. What is around every electrical cord? Rubber! What kind of suits do the men who work on electrical lines wear? Rubber!

Energy flows up from the earth through the human's chakras and out the crown and then loops back down from the Universe in a figure 8 pattern. Right handed folks receive their earth energy coming up through their left side; and they send energy out through their right side, Left handed vice versa.

Now let's add heavy tennis shoes on your feet to the mix! Hello, that's like putting your finger in the aquarium's intake filter system AND blocking everything that is supposed to be filtered out. You wonder why your wattage is decreased and not as effective! Take off those tennis shoes and you'll see a world of difference in the flow through you as a conduit!!

I suggest that you wear leather, wood or cork bottomed shoes, preferably LEATHER! Yes, you can afford them. Go to the big fancy store, find your size and fit, then buy them on internet discount shoe sites.

Rubber bottom shoes can keep you from sleeping. They create prickly feet, restless legs, leg cramps and lower back pain, because your energy is backing up and creating your own energy septic tank. Soaking your feet in water will pull the "gunk" energy out out out. That's why color changing water from a footbath is so interesting to a lot of people.

If you are tired after work, assess your methods of shielding and your detachment and delivery procedures. You are either using your own life force energy incorrectly, blocking its correct flow or not protecting yourself.

Being barefooted or in socks will allow the energy to run cleaner and have a faster delivery due to no obstruction. Thus we've eliminated another "lower wattage," "it makes me tired" cause.

Personal sensations while being an empath can diminish the total accuracy of your reading due to the fact that you will be distracted and preoccupied by dealing with those sensations and feelings within YOUR body that are the client's issues.

Plus the empath experience lowers your personal "frequency" by having to deal with the issue within your body! Instead, examine the sensations on the monitoring mechanisms of your mind's eye. That way you are watching and registering what is going on but not wasting time or energy of processing it through your body.

Exterior energies around your client can alter your client's energy so that it affects your evaluation.

Another healer's energy will look like a green or red jellyfish in your client's field. Radiation creates a cap of red energy. If a client's medication is too strong, it will produce a brown muddy sludge or just total darkness by numbing out the electromagnetics of the area controlled by the medication. Usually it's pain meds that affect the energy the most.

If the client's energy is "dirty" then all your current energy slide readings will look like they have a thin pale brown muddy membrane over it. That's why I ask the client to shower or bath before our session if possible.

Be sure a client gives you permission to enter their energy field and is not just placating this reading because someone wanted them to have this done! A "half" permission from a client creates a half baked assessment.

Personal Preparation

I usually try to schedule a MIDI first thing in the morning after my shower or after lunch so I can take time to get quiet in order to focus intensely on that client's issues.

For emergency scans, take a quick walk, sit or stand in a quiet space for about 1 minute while taking a few deep breaths. Then ask permissions, say your prayers. In about 2 total minutes you're ready for having the "action" flow. I say in my head "Ok God, I'm here to experience your awesomeness! It's show time."

Preparation for a regular appointment:
1. Take a few minutes of quiet time, get yourself balanced, centered and grounded.

2. Take off your shoes for better "flow." You can stand on a towel if you are in an area with inappropriate floors.
   Example: Hospital rooms, veterinarian examining areas
3. Protect and shield yourself with prayer so you will not take on the client's issues.
4. Have a glass of water or two handy and drink it during your reading. If you need to take a "loo" break during the reading, fill up that glass and have some more water with a few lemon drops in it to keep the headaches away.
5. Move away from computers, clocks, cell phones, iPods et al. You don't want any outside electromagnetic activity that you can control. Hospital, healthcare facilities and ICU are different, just double shield yourself and go to work!

You as Your Client

To perform a body scan or MIDI on yourself, ask to see the energy field of the vehicle your soul resides in.
State: I ask and it is my intent to see inside my hand now, to see inside my hand now, to see inside my hand now.

For about one minute, stare at the area of the hand that you want to view. Then close your eyes. An image of the area that you were looking at will come up on your mind's screen.

When you begin practicing this exercise, you may experience "raw" eyes and a frontal 3rd eye headache.
Drinking lemon juice in water or ½ cup Gatorade will help relieve those symptoms. The magnesium in chocolate will
also help.

Go about this with the same precision you do with a client, using the same interrogatories and directives and systematic approach.

Client Preparation before a Reading

First, explain to your client that you are going to have a regimented "order of go" in your reading. This insures that any body part or system is not missed in your evaluation.

Initial connection with the client's energy

Before starting the scan or MIDI, have a lightweight conversation or informal chat session with the client about all sorts of things (fun, serious and non-directed) to get a "feel" for their energy. Talk about their work, the family, and all things except the actual scan that you am preparing to do. If you sense that the client thinks the chatter is not productive, inform them that you are using this to coagulate their energy into a form that is easily readable and the conversation provides a "flavor" of their energy.

Before a MIDI (or any work)

1. Ask client's permission
2. Say preparation prayer to protect the client and you.

Preparation Prayer: Changing the words will change the results.
State: Thank you God/ Universe/ Higher Power for the Gift of _____. I ask and it is my intent to surround me, shield me, fill me and ground me with the Christ White Light (or your Higher Power.) I ask that all those energies, entities, angels and all those on the other side who're in charge of my soul's contract that serve the Christ white Light contribute to this consultation now, and all those in charge of_____'s contract come and work through me now only for _____'s highest and best good. I ask that _____ and I have no expectations for this session and have no human filters so that THY will be done and that the information and energy will be pure and not tainted. I ask that You use me, use me, use me, ONLY for _____'s highest and best good. Thank you. SO be it, it is done!

Having no expectations or filters (attitudes) is allowing your Higher Power to do what's best. Human expectations clog your information's purity. The difference between being an ordinary healer and extraordinary, is about being the conduit without human restrictions. By "not caring enough" to have expectations, you are channeling pure energy and pure wattage. When you are creating situations with your expectations and your human filters, YOU are narrowing and tainting the Universe's "all there is."

The Universe will determine everything. Don't get so caught up in a modality's techniques and your ego that you forget to be a pure channel and don't over think to "taint" the info or flow.

Client cooperation makes a scan or MIDI easier.

1. Ask the client to make notes during the session so they can ask questions later. Then you can "zoom in" on any area that they want to minutely refocus on again.
2. Concentrate on the information that you are downloading. Ask clients to remind you to look at specifics at the *end* of a section and again after the entire MIDI.

One of the most important aspects of a MIDI is to ask permission to enter your client's energy field.

If you proceed with clients who do not give permission for you to work on them, you are not connecting to pure energy. I also inform my clients that every energy worker they encounter should ask them for permission because it is not always implied just by making an appointment. Remind the client to have each practitioner detach from their energy for their safety, and explain that you will detach from their energy field when finished with your assessment.

Sometimes before a session starts, I provide an empty diagram image of a person's or animal's body on paper which allows the client to make localized notes during our session. We rediscuss areas that merit further clarification when the MIDI is over.

I explain how I deliver my evaluation and my methodology to clients who are not familiar with energy "lingo."

"The body's energy is like a theater. Each play has multiple scenes that hold a scrapbook of information about each performance period in your life. I review your past, present and future energy patterns within each scene."

I explain that I relate **every** impression I receive and see! I start with past life energy. Because MIDI addresses physical issues, I go around the emotional layer in order to get to the current physical energy system. After we have finished current health issues I address future energy.

I describe to them that the images I see present themselves in a multilayered folder of file images like walking through various curtains of energy that represent the various times in the client's life.

I explain that my mind's viewing screen, switches from view to view of a photographed area like a slide show or a video camera recording various aspects within that scenario. (Such as the different parts and aspects in a photograph of the stomach area).

I relate that medically compromised areas "light up" like fireflies in the order of medical urgency and importance for me to address. Those issues then fade off my visual field when I have given that information to my client. I explain that the best thing a client can have is a "blank screen," rather than one that twinkles!

While viewing an area, increment by increment, I ask the client to confirm that they indeed experience what I perceive in their past energy until the energy pictures get really clear. When the images are clear, I'm in present energy.

Oftentimes, a client will not immediately remember an incident that I describe in our first session. In our next session, they'll say "oh I remember I did have - in the past, just wanted to let you know."

If I have not seen a condition before, a client will hear me say: "give me more information about this issue," or "tell me what I need to know."

I also explain that if I'm not getting information or seeing anything I'll state "why am I not getting an answer?"

**The responsibility for clarity, acuity and information
is determined by the Universe
and NOT your guessing or interpretation.**

MIDI information is provided from the Universal library. Trust that information in the face of all the facts that might approximate another conclusion. Then you stand in truth. Always listen to what resonates within you.

I do not censor or reformulate or give my information on an "as needed basis." I inform my clients that I would want to know everything so that is why I tell them the exact information that I receive. I feel this practice reinforces the integrity and authenticity of the Gift channeling through me, rather than me rewriting the messages. If you rewrite, you're not being pure.

How to View the Body

Before approaching any body
State: "I ask and it is my intent to know and see what I need to know for _____ highest and best good now."
A MIDI should be viewed in quadrants on each of the four sides of the body so you don't miss anything, are more accurate and can determine the exact location of an issue that WILL show up if serious, in almost all quadrant views.
Use the positions of a clock to illustrate to the client "what I am looking at and where," so the client can create that clock on their body and you'll can be examining and discussing the same area.

How long does a MIDI take?
A full MIDI on a healthy person or a mini MIDI usually takes about 2 hours of evaluation. An average client with health issues and disorders usually takes 4 to 6 hours.
A typical MIDI takes 3 sessions, each about 2 hours long.
I had a client in an auto wreck. It took 8 hours for the MIDI and 2 hours of summation and "just for the record."
So plan your time and fees accordingly.

Start at the top of the head on the front of the face. I explain to the client that their left ear is 3 o'clock to me and that their right ear is my nine o'clock position since I am looking at them in a reverse pattern. Also alert them to the fact that since you are looking at a mirrored image, your frontal descriptions may be on the opposite side that you are describing.

View in sections or quadrants within each of the following perspectives:
Front View:
Head to eyebrow
Eyebrow to nose
Nose to Chin
Mouth
Chin to Collarbone
Thyroid
Collarbone to Sternum
Pulmonary system
Digestive system

Heart
Sternum to navel
   Liver, spleen, pancreas
   Navel to Pubic Bone
   Female or Male Reproduction system
   Urinary System
Thigh to Knee
Knee to Ankle
Ankle to Toes

Back View:
   Toes to Ankle
   Ankle to knee
   Knee to Thigh
   Buttock
   Pelvis area
   Lower back
   Thoracic back
      Kidneys
   Shoulders
   Cervical Spine
   Neck area
   Skull area

Brain: Over top
   Left and right anterior and posterior sides
   Mid brain
   Underside
Right side view:
   Top to Bottom
Left Side view:
   Top to Bottom

Side views provide invaluable information!
They let you know how far within a body and how far under the skin
the issue is located.

The Order of Viewing Energy Layers

The Framework for viewing is each stage of life.
You will see them in this order:
Past Energy I Emotional I Present I Future I Transition

1. Past energy is the first physical layer. It is thick (like a membrane) and a little murky i.e. the images are a little hazy or fuzzy. That's how you identify this energy level.

Past energy is anything that is not *today at this moment*, and including what the client did yesterday. This "old energy" blueprint will always be the foundational building block and baseline reading of **each area** that you are evaluating.

Womb,	Birth,	Infancy,	Toddler
Childhood,	Pre teen,	Adolescence	
Young adult			
Adult			
Mid life adult			
Mature adult			
Senior adult			

2. Emotional energy is the second energy tier you pass through. It looks like a Vaseline smear over each section of the client's life energy sections. It resembles a transient smear because emotional energy changes day to day, and only coagulates into a discernable diagnosable pattern in various lifetime segments. I do not read this energy level *unless* it creates a major physical dysfunction. MIDI is a physical evaluation.

3. Present or Current energy is the third layer. As you become immersed in current energy and not just transitioning into it, it is clean and in very clear focus.

4. Future energy is the last energy layer. It lies beyond the physical body and holds all of its information in a very sheer film, including Death and Transition.

+++++ The important thing to remember +++++
you will see **each** of these energy layer segments within **each** quadrant's individual sector, and then within each area, or organ or cell. It's imperative to proceed incrementally to insure accuracy.

How to See Energy

Exterior Energy
Exterior scans view the outside energy fields of the physical body called the aura.

To see the exterior field (on yourself)
1. **State:**
   I ask and it is my intent to see my energy field now,
   I ask and it is my intent to see my energy field now,
   I ask and it is my intent to see my energy field now.
2. Then close your eyes tight and say "shift energy and refocus now."
3. Open your eyes softly, try not to blink.
4. Stare at the <u>edges</u> of the subject (i.e. your shoulder line, top of your head, or the outside edges of your hand) until you see a soft glow emanating up from the area that you have chosen to read. Think the television show *Touched by an Angel* as an example.

When that glow appears, congratulations, you are looking at exterior energy (aura)! The more you practice this exercise, the quicker and stronger an aura will manifest on demand. Practice looking at your energy field in the bathroom against a plain wall in front of a mirror, or put your hand on a white sheet of paper and look at the spaces <u>in between</u> the fingers, or on the outside outline of your arm to see your aura.

Once you active this Gift, it's activated for the rest of your incarnation unless you decide not to use it.   It takes about 2 weeks to get proficient. Everyone has an aura that is readily available to be viewed. See *Hands of Light* by Barbara Brennan for aura meanings.

A MIDI examines INTERIOR energy sometimes called "interior viewing" or "inner vision." You can practice this on yourself in front of a mirror.

To See Inside the Body
1. Stare at the <u>area </u>you want to see (i.e. your shoulder, heart or hand) for about a minute or less. The more you practice the less time it will take you to observe the interior image you request to see.

2. Then close your eyes tight and say
    a. "shift energy and"
    b. "refocus now."
3. Keeping your <u>eyes closed</u>
    Ask to see the physical energy field you wish to view
    State:
    a. I ask and it is my intent to see the energy inside
       of _ (My hand) _now
or b. I ask and it is my intent to see __ (the heart) _ now.

Use your mind's eye to "see" on the inner screen of your mind. Some individuals are able to see a visual overlay of the subject area with their normal vision.

For a general body scan overview state:
1. "I ask and it is my intent to see __Client's name body now.
2. "Show me what I need to know now."
    Ask to "show me that again" if it was not clear the first time.

Energy that represents health issues
Energy spots that are aberrant from the "normal" healthy energy pattern of an area, will present as points of illumination (which to me, look like fireflies).

This "spot" or area that "lights up" is indicative of an energy area that requires immediate assessment or is an important health issue, symptom or disorder demanding high priority in your evaluation.

The Universe will continue to bring each "highlighted" issue to your attention in all viewings within each quadrant.

To determine what is going on in that area
State: I ask the Universe to give me information about this area now.
    The Universe will then download a dossier on each issue.

How to look at energy
Operate your mind's eye like a video camera viewing the various life stages and the layers in those stages.

Do <u>not</u> shift back and forth from the client's body energy to normal frequency to answer questions while you are viewing, then jump back in to view again. This will create a vibrational disturbance that usually precipitates a *major* headache! Just shift the lenses in your mind and keep looking at the "darkroom" images while you are talking to the client.

How the Energy Images Appear

My visual span is from prebirth and into the future. Every individual's energy contains a timeline that I can follow, "track," interpret and diagnose. Think of it as an ascending stairway, one step builds upon another step, and each section contains layers of sandwiched and interwoven slides. (Cells make tissue makes skin)

Transition	Purple swirl & upward spiral
Future_____	Thin filmy iridescent overlay
Present_____	Clear
Emotional_____	Cloudy Vaseline smear
Past_____	Fuzzy edged hazy images

Each image of a spot or area will appear on the screen of your mind like a stacked slide show sandwich. Once you address that area's image slice your mind will move to the next slide slice within that area or another segment of the territory being assessed.

The only way that I can move a slide presentation along, is to relate the knowledge that I have gathered from that slice to the client. Or ask them to make of note of it, in case it might be something we want to evaluate later. That way the Universe insures the client receives the "info."

Once I describe the physical size, location, condition and give my intuitive evaluation of an area to the client, that slide screen multi folder disappears and my focus shifts to the next folder or sandwich area to assess. Slices of slideshows will always move to the next slideshow after you report the results to your client.

If it is your intent to swap different layer positioning of the slices or readjust your zoom lens to review the energy layers that you're evaluating, you must ask the Universe to present the images in the reworked manner you want to view them in.
Example: "Stack the slides so I can evaluate this situation from the top." Or, "rearrange the slide slices so I can look at it from the left side "(this is good to use for Vertebrae).

Only after I have finished the entire quadrant or section, if something is "really important", do I move to the future to assess the possibility of prognosis for upcoming health events.
Example: I stated "there is a dot that should be watched over the next few years as it could be prostate cancer." In 3 years he was diagnosed with prostate cancer in that spot.

Cover future issues after you have finished the entire body.

During a follow-up scan, the initial slices that made up the first diagnostic slide presentation should be compared to the current view. **State:** I ask to see and review a slide of _____from ____'s past timeline and from _____'s current energy now.

This will allow you to understand what is currently happening and how it has changed from the past to the present.

How to Interpret Slices & Slides

My interpretation comes from looking at each slice within an energy slide's layer
1. Evaluate how it presents: ask why it's in that position
2. Evaluate the time it showed up on your "screen" and why the placement is significant

If you have a medical background, don't try to read "known" symptoms. Focus on reading and being educated by the actual energy of the client's cells, nerves, organs et al and body systems. Don't allow your education to prejudice the presentation.

When determining clarity to see if an energy pattern is in past energy, or that energy pattern's "blurriness" is information about the health issue

start in the past energy of an area,

then ask to be switched to current energy

then to future energy and then back to current energy.|
Those varying views will provide clarification as to what it is.

Use the information you initially receive rather than altering what you think as you see various changes. The minute you filter any information you are tainting the accuracy!

Another way to get greater accuracy is to ask to view the slices swapped back and forth within the same slide inside that energy layer. Ask to stack them in various combinations and ask for more information about each combination. This shuffle and restack method will furnish multiple minutia details of what is occurring.

Inform the client about EACH impression that you get with each different stacking option. Explain that you are examining different arrangements in order to derive more details. Cumulatively you'll reach a better evaluation with all the indicators the shuffle and stack method gleans.

Some practitioners tell clients information on an "as needed basis," I do not think that is a good approach. It doesn't honor the Gift of direct information your client is receiving through you as a channel. I believe that good, bad or ugly, each client has the right to the information provided and that the client can then discern WHAT to do with that knowledge. If you do not know, have a clue, or aren't sure, TELL the client exactly that! Then ask them if you can email or call them =back later after you "think about this for a while."

I had a client from Asia that was being misdiagnosed. Our reading was a very precise and accurate one. We decided that she should go to the Mayo clinic for treatment.

Throughout this entire process she would call me about once a week and ask me if I was hearing "Cancer." I NEVER got the word "Cancer." I got that she was going to be fine. I told her that if I had heard the word Cancer, I certainly would have relayed that information to her so she could discern if it resonated with her.

Multiple times she called all hours of the day and night wanting to know if it was Cancer. I assured her that I never got the word Cancer and if I did, I would tell her. I would want to know if it was me.

When she was finally thoroughly re-diagnosed at Mayo, everything that I stated about the interior physical deterioration, surgery description, post operative outcome and future prognosis and probabilities were 100 % correct and "right on" in location and size. The client then informed me "it was Cancer!"

I was furious and felt betrayed by my Guides. I had always completely believed in what they say! I decided that if I was going to get erroneous information, then I was going to quit this profession, I only wanted the truth.

I stopped consultations. A few months later this client called and asked again if I had ever heard the word Cancer for her and had I held it back so not to frighten her. I stated no and that I was no longer doing consultations due to the fact that HER information was given to me incorrectly even though every other detail, except the word Cancer, was 100% accurate including that she is now completely fine!

After I GRILLED her numerous times about how she felt about my 100% accuracy about everything but NOT on the ONE thing she feared most, she quietly said "I need to tell you something and you need to go back to work. If you had told me it was Cancer before I left, I would have considered something different and never have gone to Mayo. However since you did say everything was going to be OK, I decided to be treated. Thanks to you I am now Cancer free and in remission."

The moral is............ when the Universe/ God know that a client can't handle specific information, the Universe will NOT give that information to YOU. Trust the Universe!

I came out of that experience with an even stronger belief that the information that I am given is for the highest and best good of my client at all times! No matter what my little earthling mind thinks it knows! SO now I trust even more!!!

First Impressions for Each Specific Area

When I start to scan the first designated area, if a region is important to my evaluation it will light up like that firefly I mentioned earlier. If a zone within a quadrant lights up multiple times, it indicates that it is either VERY serious or must be addressed immediately.

Example: I was on the phone with a man. We were looking at his heart which lit up in multiple areas with extreme intensity in my initial generalized scan and again as we were working a MIDI in that area. Additionally, his heart was flickering on and off <u>between</u> segments, so I KNEW it needed attention!

He said he was sweating and felt hot. I saw his heart had multiple blockages. I told him that he must get off the phone now! Go immediately to the emergency room or call 911 and then call me later with a follow up report.

He never returned for the rest of the MIDI. I tried to contact him on multiple occasions over several months time. He lived alone and had no local family. Instinctively, I feel that he did not make it to the hospital.

Oftentimes when you have uncovered a locale with lots of health issues, the "lighting up" will be fast and furious resembling an electrical storm. Ask clients to make notes on areas that are appearing fast, to ensure you revisit it.

When you reach a conclusion about an area, it will be cleared from your screen. Then ask the Universe to go back at the end of each segment and show you anything that you have missed.
They will comply!

Once you have seen the initial energy you can revisit any area very quickly.

Another conclusion that can be drawn from an area "lighting up on numerous occasions" is that pattern may represent a future episode. If you feel that is the correct conclusion, make sure to ask the client to make note "for the record" of your observation. I asked a client to watch a section in his brain. Several years later, he suffered insufficient vascular flow to that area resulting in vertigo, unsteadiness and compromised head positioning. John Hopkins later found it on an MRI.

While "looking," I also will hear a word(s) in my head that is totally foreign. Usually it's the medical term for the image.
Write down how you think it's spelled immediately. Later look the word up in a medical dictionary. It will add direction and depth to your analysis because you'll get another "download" or intuitive impression when you have the correct medical term.

If you don't know what you're looking at, tell the client! Ask them to give you an opportunity to figure it out.

Sometimes things do not light up, this can be misleading. Bunions may not light up. Unless you direct the focus on an area like the bunion, the Universe will address what it thinks is imperative for you to evaluate by illuminating that issue! Ask the client to ask questions about any areas of their concern if you have not already addressed them. Sometimes what they think is important, the Universe does NOT consider a health issue.

Downloading Intuitive Information

Don't talk while evaluating unless you need a client's input. By asking questions to the Universe with your mind you will receive lots of details and be able to figure out a situation by stating:
1. "Tell me what I need to know now."
2. Or "Show me, show me, show me what I need to know."

Techniques to Decipher What You See

In all the years that I have been doing MIDIs, I notify my client that what I may be describing on their right side may be on THEIR left when I perform a frontal scan. It's a mirror image of what I register.

I believe it's more important to stay connected to the view's information stream than to break the connection and say "oops what I thought was on the right is really your left!" On the frontal MIDI, use whatever technique works best for you!

KNOW that the side and rear MIDI will congeal the accuracy for determining an exact location and expanded description for each issue.

Tuning in to a client's physical vibrational frequency is like tuning into a specific radio station frequency. Distance is not the obstacle. It's the bandwidth ability of the reader that determines your capacity for details.
State: I ask to see inside of _____ physical energy now!

To see into an organ
State: "Show me what I need to see in the _____, tell me the information I need to know about the _____."

Deciphering the density or solidity of an energy pattern helps to determine the fragility of that organ's health.
Example: I looked at a child's lungs.
Her left lung, although healthy had a thinner less solid energy pattern. This indicated to me it was the more fragile lung. Turns out her left lung had repeated bouts of pneumonia, and was the first lung to show signs of a chest cold etc.

Zoom Lens Method
Acting as a MRI use your mind like a zoom lens to change the position of a vision level, see a specific area closer or in a different view or angle.

Set your intent to look at the zoomed in area, rather than BE in it. I zoomed in on someone's intestines and could feel myself swirling down a nasty mass. I learned to watch from a zoom lens perspective, and to not participate which diminishes your perspective by distracting your focus.

Adjust your zoom lens perspective like a camera lens with your intent to ask, wider, closer, back out, whatever!
State: I ask and it is my intent to see_____ from this angle (or close up, or further back, or inside) now!

Remember, repeating a request 3 times produces quicker results.

Developing a Diagnostic System

Here are some generalized color diagnostic examples. Specific color coding for disorders can be found in the Encyclopedia section that follows.

In time you will develop and add your own repertoire of relevant signals, color codes and images that fit your interpretations of diseases, disorders, medical conditions and health issues. As you begin, keep a notebook of what you see and how in time, your impressions are refined and fine tuned. Use my MIDI Images as a baseline and add patterns derived from your experiences.

Each cell's vibrational frequency corresponds to the vibrational frequency of a color. *Wheels of Light* by Roslyn Bruyere and *Hands of Light* by Barbara Brennan are good sources for the color codes they determined in their work. Valerie Hunt's work also provides interesting information.

Light areas are usually current, inflammatory or chronic issues. In my references "lighted" areas are markers for issues that need immediate evaluation. Remember, it's more important to be accurate than to be quick in determining what caused the illumination.

When an area is illuminated like a blinking firefly, it provides a great deal of information. The order of "fireflies" determines how important it is to be address:
1. The first things to light up are the primary concerns within that quadrant or the entire body.
2. The light's flickering frequency creates the medical urgency. How often it occurs, when it occurs, how it occurs such as active, inactive, ongoing, intermittent

The more the light keeps showing up, in the generalized view, between segments and in the specific area, pay real close attention! (Like the man with a heart attack.) When I see constant blinking occurring, I skip directly to that segment. Only after I have identified what needs immediate evaluation, do I return to where we were.
3. The intensity of the light tells the severity of the issue

The brighter the light, the more intense the situation is.

A steadfast glow indicates an inflammation is present or it's a current ongoing active area of the disorder.

A low grade glow means chronic/ ongoing. If there is a pale orange overlay on the lighted area, it means the immune system is involved.

4. No lights
     If an area does NOT light up, the issue is not crucial or vital to the energy layer of area you are addressing.
Example: an arm rash may not show up on a Cancer client UNLESS the client asks you to look at his arm after you have been concentrating on searching for Cancer.

     Blue is pain. The intensity, thickness, blinking, and manner in which the blue layer shows up in and between each past, present and future emery layer determines:
     1. Where, how much pain,
     2. Whether it's chronic, intermittent, serious, explosive
     3. Or a single cellular memory blueprint event.
         Example: pain generated from a car wreck.
     For an event caused pain
     State: I ask to see and know what created this pain now.
     You will be shown. I was evaluating a ladies face pain that was screaming blue and had massive red holes overlaying that pain. (Many times you will be shown a pain pattern originating from past energy that moves forward and stays hovered over current energy layers.)
     I asked to see what caused these energy images. I saw my client lying on her back with a dog biting her face. When I told her this, she confirmed that she was attacked by a dog that had ripped her face open as a child.
     Dark areas represent damaged, dysfunctional or non functional areas. Dark is an indication that an organ, tissue, cell, nerve or bone is missing some or all of its electromagnetic vibrational frequency. The darker an organ or area is, the "deader" or more lifeless that energy is. Therefore it has a lower probability of regeneration or restoration. Dark colors range from slate gray to black. Examples: Scar tissue, a mole, hole in skin
     Black means that no energy is received by that cellular structure. It's a non responsive bioenergy area.
Examples: A birthmark would be black. A non active tumor would be black due to the fact that the disease (Cancer) had killed the cells (i.e. the cells no longer had an electromagnetic vibrational frequency). Any cells killed by any disease will be black. Strokes show up as dead vascular areas in the brain.

FYI a bad bruise will have a thin black overly with deep burgundy red underneath, because momentarily the tissue is non active until the bruise heels.

Numb areas have a sheer black veil over pale blue because the pale blue represent the nerve layer, and the black means it's deadened.

Navy blue appears in brain areas representing abnormalities in electromagnetic neural firings of the brain. (MS, Parkinson's).

Nerve damage is a pale blue overlay representing malfunctioning nerves such as Paralysis or nerve damage.

A client's right side showed all pale blue. Then the image would blink away and then return. Her energy pattern's behavior and color coding represented when her Multiple Sclerosis paralysis would flare up and when it would go into remission.

Orange yellow / gold involve the immune system.

Red is life force energy and also represents blood.
A deep burgundy underlay with a heavy concentration of a black overlay usually represents death to the tissue, organ, bone or entire area.   Example: If you tune into an animal whose whole body exemplifies that coloration, 99% of the time they're at the point when that part of the body can't be revived. (Like a leg crushed by a car)

If a body has this coloration and has upwardly spiraling purple energy, then that body has begun the transition process.

Outside Involvement While Viewing

When anyone asks a question or there's a follow up inquiry while I'm evaluating a region, that query initiates a separate screen specific to the question that is alongside of my first slide. Then I review the initial screens and readjust my focus by zooming in and changing the close-up lenses (like on a camera) comparing that view to the differences within the new slide. While looking at this new charted area, it triggers more downloaded details from the Universe.

I love working with healthcare professionals and a client at the same time. Their questions intermingled with my results ignite separate screen images to answer each of their questions, and each impression is more detailed and vivid than the last. That combination creates fabulously accurate findings quickly!

Other Methods of Receiving Information

Each medical intuitive has their repertoire of input.
One medical intuitive may receive their perceptions from smell,
another visualizing energy in their mind's eye or actually seeing the
organ and its energy.

My MIDI method of dissecting and creating energy slides like a
human MRI or X- ray machine is when I actually see inside the client's
body (either onsite or at a distance) their cells, nerves, bones, tissue,
organs and systems to accurately determine the location, extent, and
severity of physical problems.

I learned in a conference as some allopathic physicians call it
"anatomical intuitive medical diagnosis" is actually more accurate that
an MRI which has an approximate variable accuracy rate due to the
fact that an MRI only perceives its image from exactly where it is
aimed and is restricted to the limited position parameters of the area
imaged. Also in a MRI each disease process has a different reported
diagnostic accuracy depending on the part of the body being scanned.

An intuitive anatomical medical scan or MIDI creates a 360
degree virtual view of the specific area AND all the other areas and
positions within the condition's vicinity. So you have a 100 percent
readable area, only limited by the reader's bandwidth of frequency
ranges, and their ability to interpret and evaluate the findings
correctly.

**Hearing medical words for diagnosis is another means of
Universal downloads.** Normally when giving a consultation, I "hear"
words in my mind that I have NO idea how to spell. So I pronounce
them out loud to the client. We then locate the word or as close as
possible in a medical dictionary. I instruct the client to ask the
healthcare provider about that word in relation to their health issue.
The physician knows exactly what to rethink, retest or re-observe.

Usually that unknown medical verbiage is the exact condition or
anatomical descriptive area or medical technical word for the health
issue, energy area, or presenting disorder. I suggest that you do not
dismiss, this added information even if you cannot identify it in your
personal vocabulary.

Sometimes when you are reviewing the *Human Anatomy* book,
you'll flip a page and there will be a word whose spelling audibly
pronounced will have matched the word you "heard" through your
clairaudient intuition. Be sure you also get a *Taber's Medical
Dictionary* so you can look up and understand disorders.

Some practitioners including myself use their hands for an additional dimension of intuitive diagnosis with an onsite client. How is this done?

> Rub your hand together to stimulate nerve ending receptors.
> Enter the client's energy field at 45 degree angle.
> Hold your hand over the area your want to scan with the palm down.
> Spread your fingers apart to give you greater information and nuances.
> Take the same hand and go over the same area using the back side of your hand for additional information.

The sensory codes for using your hands:
> Heat indicates pain.
> Blowing cold energy at your hand indicates infection.
> Thick energy is a blockage.
> Pulsating energy represents aberrations in a healthy energy field. Then look inside and "see" what it is.

Smelling is another form of subjective diagnosis.
I know a man who can smell death approaching. So don't discount any additive input. No informational delivery system is more important than another.

Dreams can be great information tool. This Prayer can help to interpret dreams and the knowledge contained within them.
State: "I ask and it is my intent to be shown in clear ways that I can understand as a human, the knowledge and information that I need to know for my highest and best good and for the highest and best good of my client."

Some practitioners think it's safe to go searching for answers at night during sleep. When you wake up in the morning, are you tired from working in the astral planes throughout the evening? Do not leave your body and astro travel. This is dangerous. You will attract unwanted entities and energies that will attach to you and your sliver cord. Do not leave you body. Set your intent that your energy does your work, in a protected shielded cocoon.

There are many intuitive healers who have a normal structured "day" job and work for the Universe at night. If that's you, keep your day job! Use this prayer:
State: "I ask and it is my intent for my soul to stay in my body, and for my energy to do the work where it is needed. So be it, it is done!"

Presenting Findings to Your Client

The best finding for a client is to have a blank screen; however that is rarely the case. The second best thing is for you to take your time, and tell EXACTLY what you receive and let the client determine how to handle the information.

Example: When I first looked at my client, her body lit up like those running Christmas tree lights. There were little dots going all over around and through her body's energy system in plastic clear tubing during my initial quickie overview. I had NO idea what that was and told her. I knew this was going to be interesting!

Of course I LOVE hunting down what is wrong! SO I started grilling the Universe, "show me what I need to know, tell me what I need to know now" all the while watching this profound very active, highly moving light show!

I heard the word Leukemia. I studied her "light up" phenomena again, and heard Leukemia............ I told her that I did not want to upset her, but I was obligated to my Gift to let her know that I was continuously hearing the word Leukemia, and that I think the little lights were Cancer traveling in her blood. She quietly stated "I was diagnosed with that yesterday at the Mayo Clinic and just wanted a second opinion."

Always inform your client that you have not seen what you are looking at ---if you have not seen a particular situation before. It maintains your integrity to the information that you are acquiring. It lets your client know that you are taking your time to gather the information and are examining it for content in order to determine the cumulative findings.

Future Energy Issues: Identification & Diagnosis

Because the human energy field contains all information, future energy prognostics are available to the medical intuitive who has the capacity to tap into future energy thinner higher range bandwidth frequencies. Your consultations are just as valuable even if you only read current energy.

Most of my clients have had future cancer metastases diagnosed by me before they registered on a MRI. The reason a medical intuitive reading can provide this additional information is because in addition to the physical body's energy file, you also have the human energy field that surrounds the physical body. In medical intuitive diagnosis, this separate energy layer over the physical body's energy provides another entirely different area for diagnosis and prognosis.

Diseases and disorders first appear in the exterior energy field BEFORE entering the actual physical field. Thus a forthcoming heart attack, infection, cancer, nerve damage, ruptured blood supply, pulmonary event, impending disease or even a simple sore throat registers as a hovering grey energy above and apart from the specific energy of a physical body part. Think of the future informative energy resembling a cloud hovering over a specific part of the earth before its going to become absorbed into and affect that location.

The medical inituitive's ability to identify that "black cloud of health issues" and to assess the timeline it will manifest into the physical body, will provide an invaluable evaluation for the client.

Future prognosis can help determine if an intervention (i.e. changing lifestyle, eating habits or adding another current treatment) can affect the outcome, or a "heads up" on monitoring a health issue that might be eliminated with appropriate medical vigilance. Additionally a future energy scan can provide information that will become "known" at a later date.

I had a client with ongoing bladder cancer that was removed on several occasions. When I scanned his urinary system, I informed him that the bladder was not the origin source of the cancer. Instead the active area that was continuing to produce cancer cells that grew in his bladder was located at the base of his right kidney where it attached to the ureter and that he should have an MRI of that area. It was also my assessment that only upon removal of the area in his lower kidney would his physicians be able to contain and obliterate any further cancer outbreaks in his bladder lining.

Every time he would get a new cancerous growth and have new MRI images made, those films showed nothing, I continued to urge him to keep monitoring and MRI-ing that area. I received his phone call later telling me that FINALLY the area I had described years earlier had shown up on the MRI and his physician was going to address it. With proper treatment, medication and vigilance, he no longer has recurrences.

With Cancer metastases, future energy scans can save a lot of time under certain circumstances. I had a client that was ONLY going to have a specific spinal bone area irradiated. I urged her to get the radiologist to re MRI her again before they waited another 6 months to see how their current radiation regime worked. Fortunately, they redid an MRI and found new metastases had spread to the hip bone area in addition to the bottom of her spine. She was able to address all the metastases with a revamped radiation treatment and had much better results than waiting 6 months while those areas I had identified, would have been left untreated.

Additional Information
after Evaluating the Physical Energy

When you have finished your physical reading, I suggest that you get the book of actual bodies used in most medical schools *Human Anatomy* to look up and compare what you saw to the factual anatomical feature. Then give your client the medical terminology, location and proximity to other organs or inner recognizable tissues, bones et al, so they can furnish that additional information to their healthcare provider for further discussion, testing, or monitoring.

You can also draw your perception of the location of an issue and provide that to the healthcare provider so they can take it to the MRI, CT, MUGA or Ultra sound operator and "aim for that" area. Did you know that the film's findings are only as good as the directives of the the the technician's aim at the "spot," the age of the machine's technology (new, used or old) and their "reading of the results?" If the focus beam is off a nano meter, your healthcare provider can miss an issue. That's the value of 360 degree MIDI.

I fractured 5 vertebrae and three radiologists did not register it on their films. After the first MRI, the radiologist said their "might be the slight risk of a fracture." And how old was that machine! When I asked my physician to retake the lateral spinal view because it was taken from the wrong angle, he said "don't worry, it won't make that much difference." How about 3 fractures worth! I changed physicians!

After I suggested WHERE the new physician's technicians aim the beam, they "discovered" 3 fractures that were not revealed earlier due to the positioning of the machine and angle of penetration for imaging by that community college intern. The MOST frustrating thing of all, I could see where they were, and had to "work with the traditional medical system" to be treated. Even I have to deal with "the System."

Another incredible source of information that sparks your intuitive process is an Internet search. I always look up the diseases, disorder and issues that the client presents. If something "triggers" my mind after scanning the information, then I ask my Guides "what do I need to know."

Often times when I'm trying to uncover the underlying cause for an illness that no one can determine or diagnose, I keep looking up and researching words that come to my mind that relate to the images that I've viewed. If something sparks my interest I read along those lines. If it doesn't resonate with me I keep scanning and gleaming through information until something strikes a chord with me.

If your research produces something that resonates with you as a major contributing issue, read and listen, read and listen and ask. This research will educate you and tune in and refine your intuitive diagnostic abilities while viewing the client.

The MIDI will allow you to "know" how to set your intent and how to focus your research approach on the condition to be evaluated. Keep refining your slide images and zooming in an out of the various bodily systems and researching what you "see." This will provide a clear stream of symptoms that all add up to a high percentage of correct diagnosises and is especially helpful in keying your intuition to discover a diagnosis for very rare diseases.

FYI, the process of re-examining slides from your client's reading and researching the Internet with words, or trying to describe what you saw as a symptom, will take HOURS, I mean HOURS to redefine and further revisit layer upon layers of images and intuitive perceptions that individually spark yet ANOTHER set of intuitive keys to discovery. Personally, I LOVE those "hunting adventures" when my cumulative findings become invaluable and life changing for my client's health journey.

MIDI Conclusions & "For the Records"

After I have finished reading the client's body, I ask if there are any final questions, areas or systems that they want me to re-examine at a more in depth level than our initial view.

If so, go back to that area's original screen and ask to specifically see a more detailed view than the initial image. If nothing changes, then your primary assessment was all there is to know about that particular region.

After all random questions and everything is addressed including whatever they want to revisit in *Human Anatomy* or *Taber's Medical Dictionary* or rediscuss with other information, I present a **"for the records" summation**.

This is a cumulative summary of the highlights of what you discovered, discussed and the order of go in which each current health issue needs to be addressed and what should be closely monitored.

Last but not least, be sure you completely disconnect and detach from each client's energy field after your evaluation.

At the end of every consultation, I say always say "Thank you for my Gift." Then I analyze what the client taught me and examine how I can be better for the next client.

Pediatric MIDI

A pediatric MIDI is like adult viewing; however, a child is more sensitive to your energy permeating their energy field as are animals. DO NOT forget to ask permission as they are souls to and be sure to have their parents or legal guardian sign the consent forms.

Don't be too hasty in identifying an issue, as undeveloped growing organs bones et al. are processing, and that transitional energy requires even more exacting and detailed observations because it is not as "set" as adult energy.

A Few More Things worth Mentioning

Hypochondriacs

This group of individuals needs to be mentioned, because invariably you will have them as your client. They will not show physical energy patterns of medical disorders. However their emotional layers will predominate in presentation over their physical energy fields.

Although I can read emotional energy layers, I do not choose to do so. I enjoy physical issues much more so I focus my practice on doing that kind of evaluation. After I assure them that I see no physical issues, I suggest to the Hypochondriac "perhaps you should consult a professional that deals with emotional issues."

If you want to give a reading on both issues, do a MIDI first and then the emotional scan so your MIDI images won't be "filtered" or distorted by the emotional energy layer. Then you can combine the knowledge for the clients greater good

There are people experiencing physical issues that manifest from emotional issues and are not hypochondriacs. This group genuinely has physical issues and wants to rule out major disease, disorders et al.

A woman came to me with severe back and leg pain although x-rays, myleograms showed nothing. After evaluating her, I agreed that there was no physical cause for her debilitating pain. However, as I explained to her, upon examination I did see a huge gray smudge of emotional energy over her heart. I felt she had recently suffered a huge emotional heartfelt trauma which was creating her lower back and leg pain. She confided two weeks prior, her son was killed. Bingo!

She left our consultation feeling better knowing that her physical pain was manifested from authentic emotional trauma and would resolve without surgery et al. I also suggested that she investigate grief counseling to help her handle and resolve the issues that were reeking havoc with her nervous system.

Amount of Time to Safely View Each Client

I suggest that you keep viewing to no more than 2 hours at a time, and take a midway break. Drink plenty of water WHILE reading your client. Occasionally you will have a headache or nausea if you extend your reading's timing beyond your body's threshold for holding a different vibration.

It's in YOUR best interest to have multiple sessions rather than a long one. As soon as the information does not flow immediately or the images start getting fuzzy, you need to end and schedule another session.

If you are really tired, your screen will go blank or you will not be able to discern the various layers. This condition will destroy your accuracy.

Here are few tidbits:

Hair and nails grow faster when you are doing scans.

Headaches clear up with about a half cup of pedialyte.

If you stay in a session too long you may use up too much magnesium and have a craving for chocolate.

After a consultation meat will ground you.

Follow-up and Recheck Body Scans

If a client requests a "follow up" to monitor their condition, recheck a procedure or treatment or as an annual physical assessment, that "follow up" MIDI begins with the last image that my mind's eye recorded in their "file."

Ask to see their current energy impressions and overlay their original energy or create a side by side display that allows you to see if any change has occurred. This can be done for years!

Part 3

Trust the information given to you by your Higher Power and Guides

The Encyclopedia of Bioenergy Patterns That Identify Diseases, Disorders & Health Issues
(Encyclopedia of Bioenergy Patterns coming in 2011)

The following bioenergy patterns were given to me by God/ the Universe and have been an extremely accurate diagnostic energy language for me. I offer these patterns to you in simplistic descriptions that you can relate to. Hopefully the image descriptions illustrate the concepts in a manner you can readily understand.
I tried to paint their picture with my words.
Remember, these concepts are seen in my mind's eye with my eyes closed. I rarely perform an onsite MIDI. If I initiate an onsite MIDI, I look at the client, then close my eyes and see the image of the area come up in my mind first before it overlays the viewing area. Therefore my encyclopedia of descriptions is what I see inside my mind.
The listings, in alphabetical order on the left, represent the disorder.
Also in the left column is the disorder and the way the slices are stacked within the energy pattern's slide.
Corresponding on the right side is the energy pattern's description. Each of these descriptions represents multiple layers of energy slices superimposed over the area or organ, bone, tissue, nerve system (you get the idea) that you are viewing.
What you are sensing will be areas where the energy actually looks or the slides and slices subtly look and feel "different." The textures and multiple combinations of each energy slice create the diagnostic "differences" and is what I have described.
Everyone's interpretation of recurring energy pattern coloration tends to be consistent with the specific vibrations that make up each color's frequency bandwidth. However the medical intuitive must have the ability to see and evaluate that vibrational frequency.
It is of utmost importance that you understand that each energy layer's (past, present or future) slides and slices are located on top of the actual organ, bone, intestine, blood vessel or nerve ganglia etc. as it looks in the *Human Anatomy Book.*
Think of this language like multiple layers of transparent tissue and then within each transparent tissue an entire image substructure of more multilayered tissues that are placed over each anatomical object.

I do not know human anatomy, unless and until it's while I'm viewing or channeling. The upside is that I go into a reading totally clean with no preconditioned images, ideas or medical background that creates any preconceived ideas or conclusions.

I start with a blank screen and blank ideas of what is going to be presented within each body. Everything, fact, image, and what I receive and intuitively perceive from that information is given to me as I perform a MIDI session for the body itself.

If you do not believe there is a Higher Power, medical intuitive diagnostic imaging™ will definitely confirm to you that there is! I always feel as if I am going to a wonderful party when I start a MIDI session. I get to show up and watch the "presents" present themselves.

Due to the fact that I receive the knowledge as I am relaying that information to the client, I feel as IF I am opening a present from the Universe, to Gift those facts to the client. I am always in awe of what is unfolding to me and being made aware through me to each client.

Here's Framework and order of go in my viewing.
My coding for the descriptions following:
PE- Past Energy Layer has a fuzzy and hazy thin to thick quality depending on the activity in that layer.
CE- Current Energy layer is clear viewing and tells it like it is!
FE- Future Energy Layer is very sheer and changes its translucency according to what will be occurring.
A few more things to remember in regards to these images:
1. If you have a medical background, don't get caught up trying to read symptoms.
2. You are reading the actual energy patterns as told to you by the language of the disease within a person's organs & body systems.
2. The Encyclopedia represents Current Energy; however each can take place in the Past or Future layer view

Composition of an energy pattern slide (EPS).
Each slice **(S)** constructs and contributes to the total energy slide's **(EPS)** diagnosis. **Example:**

Bladder Infection **EPS** = Yellow **S**/ Orange **S** Bladder wall	A bladder infection will show as a yellow orange area on the corresponding wall where the infection is located.

A	

Abscess
 	
    Red
    Gold
    White
	An abscess always has a bright white inner center encapsulated by a light gold emanating outward surrounded by an angry red flamed edge.

Aches
 	
    Blue
    Area
	Aches are sheer cellophane slices in varying shades of blue over the affected area. The shade of blue determines the intensity. The action of the blue slide in the various layers determines when it happened and how long the ache has and will occur.

Acne
 	
    Skin
    Yellow white
	Acne is a red pothole in the skin's surface. In PE it looks like burgundy smudges. In CE it is either under the skin's cellular structure or sitting on the edge with a tiny yellow white glow penetrating the area's surface.

Addictions	Addictions permeate the entire PE, CE or FE layers like a huge grey brown Vaseline smudge comparable to emotional energy. Addiction energy shows up in the energy layer of origination with the symptoms in the organs and affected systems. The symptoms change in each P, C or F energy layer as the addiction manifests it's destruction within each of the body's systems.
Adrenal Problems	Show up as little almonds above the kidneys. Gray if they are sluggish and swollen burgundy if they are overworked. It's my opinion that this is the current catchall for problems that can't be identified. I have had multiple clients come to me with

	adrenal problems and in my sight, there was nothing wrong physically! Malfunction does show up in energy!
Aging	Aging energy fields are just less clear than CE. The factual presentation of aging shows up in each specific bodily system with its own set of" wear and tear" factual symptoms and shapes. Ex: an aged bladder looks like a sagging bladder in CE.
Aids	Presents a massive overflow of golden, ochre glow over all the energy layers affected at its onset. Then each symptom creates its own specific slide pattern of dysfunction in the systems affected.
Alcoholism	see Liver
Allergies	I do not see what creates the allergic reaction. I do see where and how the body responses to the allergic trigger such as swelling, closed bronchial tubes, etc.
Alzheimer's Disease Navy Black Brain	Creates a navy blue with black undertone haze over the affected area of the brain.
Amnesia Gray Brain	Is a literal "fog" slate gray area over the brain during the energy timeframe in which it occurred.
ALS (Lou Gehrig's' Disease) Amyotrophic lateral Sclerosis	ALS does not present as an entire disease. It depicts various symptomatic slide patterns in the affected organs and body function systems. You have to put the

	cumulative read of all afflictions together to discern ALS.
Anemia	The blood looks dark burgundy and feels heavy while the skin appears jaundiced for severe cases.

Ankles
  Weak
      Pale amber
      Ankle
	Weak ankles demonstrate a pale gold amber glow within the affected areas and on the exact site of the tendon, muscle and ligament energy layer.

Anus
  Fistula
 	
      White gold
      Orange
      Red
      Fistula
	Anal fistula is a line from the inner body core energy to the outside of the rectum in a dark burgundy, coated interiorly with a bright light gold. At the anal opening area, it is like a pimple, and if infected is a burning orange gold surrounded by plump pale red energy.

Anus
  Hemorrhoids
      Burgundy
      Navy red
	Hemorrhoids look like an egg drop with the outside ages in an angry red burgundy with a throbbing inner layer of navy red.

Anus
  Itching
      Yellow
      Red
      Anus
	Anal itching appears as a bumpily yellow to denote current activity, with a red underlay indicating agitated subcutaneous capillary agitation.

Anus Rectal Bleeding	Is a pulsating blood red off and on energy pattern appearing in the energy layer in which it occurs.
Appendectomy	Solid black image of the removed organ.

Appendicitis Light gold Deep gold Red Appendix	The appendix is a throbbing red and deep gold organ with pale light gold overlay energy. The intensity of the overlay determines the degree of infection.
Arteries	Only show up if they are damaged. Depending upon the affliction, the arteries show different colored energy patterns that will determine their diagnosis.
Arthritis Gold Red Bone or joint	Is pale gold inflammation energy over the damaged area. It has a sheer red edge hear the bone.
Asthma Gray mesh Lung	Is a patchy pale gray smoky smooth mesh over the affected lung area. The darker the energy the worse the asthma. If the aforementioned layer also has a sheer red layer, it means bleeding within the lung tissue, gold overlay indicates infections and a purple spot is the beginning of areas that left unattended could become cancerous.
Athlete's Foot	Looks like crusty white patches over the skin.
B	
Back Disc Herniated	Herniated disc looks like a black tire lying on its side with the good area of the disk medium gray to clear. The black area is herniated and non functioning.
Back Slipped disc	A slipped disc will light up and show misalignment by the direction of its displaced energy.

Back
    Cervical spine
 	
    Skin
    LIGHTED area
    Damage pattern
	The spine will light up with a spotlighted area when there is damage. The cervical spine is as intense as the lower spine, yet presents its energy pattern just under the skin's surface. The "damage" will be a separate energy pattern.

Back,
    Vertebral
    Fracture
	The cracked vertebrae area is black while the rest of the intact vertebrae has a smoke grey edge.

Balance, Loss of Vertigo Inner ear	Vertigo lights up the inner ear, The affected nerve area has an overlay of intermittent heavy dark energy that splays out like the spokes of a wheel.
Bile Duct Obstruction	Looks like a shiny straw through the liver with very delineated edges.
Blacking Out	Blacking out shows brain area energy firing then suddenly going off the screen. Like a short circuit in a cable transmission on a TV. During a black out, the brain loses its electromagnetic continuous connection and the active energy layer disappears.
Bladder Incontinence	The physical bladder energy is a complete pale cinnamon charcoal energy that has an extremely pale gray moving stream of inconsistent energy thru the exterior outlet that doesn't stop even when you move to another organ. If there is inflammation from the inconstancy, the exterior opening is pale red, and you can see the drip energy pattern

Bladder Infection Yellow orange Bladder	A bladder infection will show as a yellow orange area on the corresponding wall where the infection is located.
Bladder Tacked	In a bladder that has had surgery and is "tacked" up, the sutures highlight and look like upside down staples. The top area is a wavy elastic stacked area (think sagging socks) with the top area sutured to the top of the bladder cavity wall.
Bladder Spasm Blue or red Rumpled bladder	The floor of a bladder that spasms or creates extreme urgency has a rumpled floor, like the surface of bubble paper. Spasms look like off and on mixed red and blue spike patterns.
Bladder Weak	A weak bladder demonstrates a lower edge that lies like a spent balloon against the bladder wall. It has no discernable height, since it does not hold its shape on the edge of the weakened area.
Blood Cancer	See Leukemia
Blood Pressure	Ask to see the vascular system. Any areas that are darkened are areas that are not holding a steady vascular pressure. Then zoom in to determine the cause which will be separate slide.
Bleeding	Looks like a large throbbing red burgundy gellulous blob over the area that is active. If the bleeding has

	stopped, the "blob" will have a black sheer veil over it and will be stagnant.
Bleeding Gums	Have a burgundy red seepage from the area that meets with the tooth and will present intermittently.
Blisters Blue Pale Gold Red Skin	The actual blister outline shows with a pale gold glow dome while the inner edge meeting healthy skin is fire red. Over all of this is a veil of blue varying in intensity to determine the pain level.
Bloating Gas	Looks like a sheer whitish pale gray cumulus cloud hovering over the affected area.
Blood Clot	see Embolism
Blood Vessels in the Brain	Healthy blood vessels in the brain will not show up on your screen, unless you set your intent to seen them. However, crimped rumpled (think wires) navy energy represents a problem with the vascular system in the brain.
Bone Marrow Cancer	Bone marrow cancer looks like dark brown and black leopard spots within the defined bone area. If they are dark red, some of the affected area is still live tissue.
Bone Fracture Blue Black line White indicator Bone	A bone fracture looks like a black magic marker line drawn to delineate where the break is. On top of that is a blue layer that determines the pain level and at the end of the broken bone is bright white to indicate

	extreme abhorrent activity.
Brain Damage Navy Brain	Dark areas of navy blue in brain tissue indicate that there is less electromagnetic activity which means a decrease of function in those areas controlled by that portion of the brain. Any area that's fires up a spike of white determines where the origin of the "disconnect" is, unless it's an overall cellular outage caused by a disease. That disease will provide its symptoms in the affected areas so you can deduce a diagnosis.
Brain Aneurysm Stroke Navy Burgundy Charcoal Brain	A stroke area is dark navy, with ruptured blood vessels in deep burgundy. All non functioning vascular systems have a black interior with a deep burgundy outside edge. The charcoal pattern over the brain area determines the degree of cellular damage. The darker the brain matter the less probability of regeneration.
Brain Bleed from over thinned blood	A brain bleed shows up as a dark burgundy very sheer (think hose) helmet over the brain, with a light source in the initial area where the bleeding occurred.
Brain Cancer	Brain cancer illuminates where each tumor is located. Then you inspect each tumor to determine the cancer's degree of tissue invasion. Dead tissue is black, either in a complete tumor or on the area within each tumor or on the dead edge of a tumor. Most have bright white outlines of the tumor (think egg yolk) with edges of

	extreme orange. The active growing edge area is like a solar flare of red and white and varying gold. A benign tumor can be almost black and a serious tumor can be black. Be VERY careful and detailed in your observations.
Brachial Plexus Nerves	If the brachial plexus nerves are affected you will feel a deep slate gray chest heaviness in the upper chest cavity under the pectoral muscles.
Breast Calcifications	Appear as pinpoint or sized to scale bright lights with a gray edges and have a knotty appearance like cottage cheese.
Breast, Fibrous Tissue	The interior of the breast looks like a grey steel wool pad and is very dense.
Breast Tumor	Breast tumors look like hard edge yolks that are black and may or may not have an active growing edge. By doing a 360 analysis, you can determine their depth and position. Benign breast tumors look like a dark gray granular polyp and do not have intensity to their energy.
Bronchial Tube Problems with	Show up as pale blue gray tubes if they have active disorders. The sheerer the energy film the less problematic the area is. This is common in people who have sinus drips, low grade controlled asthma, or bronchitis in their medical history.

Bronchial Tube Scarring	Scarring looks like a black rumply washboard in the bronchial tubes. I had a client that had a breathing tube penetrate through her tube. It looked like a thin black hole with back flaps.
Bronchitis	Bronchitis is a crusty woolly rusty burgundy grey smudge within each bronchial tube where it is affected. Asthmatic tubes are different because asthma creates a swollen smooth energy pattern.
Bowels	see Intestines
Bruise see also Hematoma	Looks like a flattened burgundy blue black pancake within the energy field. The black is on top of the burgundy.
Burn	Burned skin looks like tight silver beige stretched to the max, melted sheer plastic. It has a bright red blue fame edge with an outer layer of pale yellow and white.
Bursitis	Looks like a jagged saw edge bulge that impedes movement.
C	
Cancer Active	The active side of cancer energy looks and is colored like a solar flare edge. The metastasizing growing edge of a cancer cell is gold yellow with an orange red jagged edge pointing in the direction that the cancer is expanding. Note: a cell could have only one side that is active while the rest of the cell is smooth edged and non active black.

Cancer in
  Brain fluid
  Spinal fluid
	Looks like bright white floating glitter that has a dark chocolate center.

Cancer
  Lung
	Lung cancer is a bright gold spot in the affected tissue. Pneumonia or an infected lung area differs from a lung cancer spot by having a cool pale blue purple edge.
	    If the cancer area is active it is surrounded by edges like an erratic fire flame of bright orange and a whiter gold on the "growing side."
	    A non growing or inactive cancer tumor has a thick banana peel skin of dark gray that can have an open active side.
	    By discerning which side of the cancer is flame or peel, you can determine where and when each cancerous growth might be "in remission," or has an actively metastasizing future potential, and the direction of that growth.

Cancer Metastases	A cancer metastasis looks like the pale white filmy webbing that is used at Halloween to mimic a spider web. The metastasis energy is sheer, has no sheen and overlays the area that is being affected. Within that metastasis, there is a center area that is bright gold with a burning flame red edge which is where the metastasis originates.
Cancer Port or Shunt	A port scar looks like a long black string bean with a silver gray outer edge.

Cancer Tumor Wrapped around	A cancer tumor that has wrapped around another organ, blood vessel, artery, etc, will appear with flame red orange yellow bright active edges and will look like moving trees roots engulfing the affected area.
Cancer Vaginal	Vaginal cancer has beige spongy hamburger areas with outer edges trimmed in pale rust.
Candida	Candida is a beret of flat red inflamed energy with a pale thin outer edge of light yellow gold to iridescent clear.
Carpel Tunnel Syndrome	Carpal tunnel is a burst of intermittent purple blue energy with a red inner core that sprays up the affected arm and spikes and swirls down into the fingers.
Cataracts	Look like blue gray medium dense see-through Frisbees overlaying the eyes.
Cerebral Palsy	Shows as each of its various symptoms, and all has a medium pale murky blue gray overlay on all the areas affected by this disease.
Cardiovascular Blocked Arteries	Present as spiking bright blue energy with an outer edge of bright gold white. Its dark burgundy purple at the blockage.
Chemical Energy i.e. Medicine	Energy that is created by medicine leaves a dark chocolate black smudgy cover over the area controlled by the meds.

Cirrhosis	Cirrhosis of the liver presents like a wire mesh (imagine steel wool ball) over the liver area that is affected. The intensity and depth of that steel wool overlay and how it's interwoven into the depth of the liver determines where and how "bad" the liver's function is traumatized.
Coccyx Broken Tailbone	The coccyx lights up a bright white gold then blue. A broken tailbone is a bright dark burgundy purple triangle at the end of the spine.

Coccyx
   Sensitive
   Tailbone
	The tailbone that has received repeated trauma, yet never broken will have a pale light sky blue purple overlay that flashes on an off to indicate intermittent yet chronic sensitivity.

Constipation Bearing Down	Looks like black clouds resting like a pool at the end of the anal rectum area with a weighted pressing down area like the bottom of a heavy bean bag.
Constipation Bowel Compaction	Compaction is several inches thick dark slate gray chocolate black overlaying intestines. Feels solid.
Colic	Presents an intermittent clenching energy that pulsates between royal blue purple edged in white white and deep red.
Coronary Thrombosis	Is a ball of bright royal blue encapsulated in deep purple burgundy inside the affected artery.

Cough
   Excessive or
   Chronic
	Excessive coughing presents as an amber gray haze over the lungs that feels undulating that is created by light pulsations or heavy bursts of energy.

Cough Light	A light cough or intermittent ongoing tickle in the throat presents as a pale smoky gray undulating, then spastic intermittent energy overlaying the area of the throat that is affected.
Cramps	Show up as clenching and unclenching energy in varying shades of blue and navy overlay.
Crown and Bridges	Show up as a dark non functioning base with a pale very sheer bluish gray overlay over the gum where they are installed.
Croup	see Bronchitis
Cuts	see Wounds
Cystitis	Is red and pale gold flamed inner liner energy over the inside of the bladder wall.
D	
Deafness,	see Ear
Death Energy	Is clear blue purple spiral swirling upward energy.
Dementia	Dementia and mental fog look liked dark gray gauze over darkest navy brain tissue.

Diabetes	Lights up the pancreas which looks either irregular bumpy navy red sometimes with yellow bald spots or more shriveled and navy blue.
DNC	A current DNC presents as red energy overlaying within the uterus that rotates inward and spins like it is going down a drain. An old DNC presents as a dark charcoal area of scarred tissue.
Disc Herniated	Herniated disc looks like a black tire laying on its side, with a "blow-out" section.
Dizziness Vertigo	Manifests as pale blue sporadic haze over the inner ear tube. Then dark gray cloud hovering over and around the outer ear. You can feel the whirling.
Dry Eye	Has deep murky gray gold film in the tear duct.
E	

Ear
    Pressure
    Blockage
	Ear pressure can be determined by mentally moving a pale white light throughout the ear tube and drum. You can determine the blockage where the energy is repelled.
	    The amount of blockage is determined by the time it takes for your energy beam to build up at the blocked area, and the heaviness of the backwashed energy.

Ear Ache	A lighted area appears where the ear is compromised. The more intense the lighted area, the greater the degree of inflammation or infection.

Eczema	Patches of taupe beige where scaling is. It looks like pitted energy in the subcutaneous layer of the physical energy.
Edema	Looks like a sheer grey white puffy overlay and feels fluid filled.
Emphysema	Is dark navy red charcoal gray clotted energy within the lungs.
Embolism Blood Clot	An embolism is a dark black tangled mass spot surrounded by a deep burgundy red edge where the actual clot is lodged. A charcoal gray mass/ area filters out around the initial dark mass and creates a secondary over layer slice that represents the physical area involved.
Encapsulation	If an area has a fine dark blue black line on the outer edge, it usually means that the encompassed area is encapsulated and not relating to the surrounding physical energy. Examples can be seen in a benign cyst, an encapsulated brain or breast tumor. The interior is like a multilayer cake. Each layer illustrates another aspect of the physical area inside the encapsulation telling its own story about what disease is involved, what tissues are affected and the various health issues currently experienced or being created. A simple example: the edge of a blister would have this line with an inflammation area inside. Various Cancerous tumors are more complex.

Endometriosis	Is a tangled charcoal gray brillo pad with a palpable thickness and depth which represents the size of the endometriosis. Its shape, depth and location are how you are able to determine how much of the uterus is involved. If a DNC has been performed in the past that energy looks like a flat dark slate gray area around the area that was biopsied.
Epilepsy	Is a dark navy blue energy in the brain tissue that is affected. It sparkles erratically which denotes abhorrent electromagnetic energy.
Epileptic Seizure	Has a purple white upward spike edged in red yellow which precedes the seizure. It becomes an erratic horizontal purple then gold spiked edgy emission from the top of the head once the seizure onset begins.
Emotions Depth	Emotional layers determine where the correlated damage manifests into the physical energy.
Esophagus, Bartlett's Disease	An esophagus that has Bartlett's at the connection of the esophagus into the stomach is inflamed and has a scarlet red scalloped edge trimmed in pale white pink gold.
Eyes, Trouble Focusing	The eye socket will have a marbleized blue beige overlay on the affected area.
Extraction	Extractions look like deep red black rotating balls of light that show up

	then spiral up and float out of your viewing field. This is the life force energy of the viewed area leaving. It will show up for teeth, miscarriages, hysterectomies, etc.
F	
Facelift	Looks like a mask where the face was changed and shows the pale gray scars feathered in the areas that were surgically altered. The skin's energy shows a shift to the direction that the face was lifted as does a neck lift.
Freckles or Birthmarks	Freckles, moles, birthmarks appear on the skin's surface energy as flat dark dime thin non functioning areas.
G	
Gall Bladder	Is angry red and swollen bumply energy slide.
Glaucoma	Looks like a pale grey sky blue contact lens over the eye.
H	
Head Trauma	Deep blood red overlay for entire head area, heavier on the side that the trauma occurred, and deep purplish black where the greatest impact was.
Heart Attack	Is a vivid lighting blue bolt surrounded by white and a strong inner purple core only in the area affected.
Heart Healthy	Is a regular medium hunter green. Most likely it will not show up on the screen at all.

Heart Healthy with Emotional Event	Hunter green heart with a haze of smoke grey encircling the entire organ rising from the heart. Think campfire smoke.
Heart Slow beat	A heart on beta blockers looks like a pumping heart grayed a bit and throbbing in a heavy slowed motion.
Heart PVC or Delayed Beat	Pale slate gray tight spongy area over the affected chamber that hiccups on and off your visual screen.
Heart Arial Fibulation	Has a layer of gray mesh screen that you can see through over the sinus node area. The degree of matting within the meshing determines the seriousness of the arterial fibulation.
Heart Arrhythmia	Is a gray mesh area (think steel wool pad)
Hematoma	A large hematoma looks like a deep burgundy blue water balloon alongside the damaged area.
Heartburn	Is an orange red swollen energy within the area in which it occurs.
Hemorrhoids	Hemorrhoids are dark red masses indicative of their size and location in the anal area. The degree of current irritation whether active or passive is determined by the amount of bright orange yellow energy above that anus. The oranger, the more infected. The yellower, the more pronounced itching. The redder/pale gold intensity indicates how much current inflammation.

Hepatitis	Shows up like a screen of steel gray burgundy over the liver. The denser the weave, the worse the dysfunction.
Hernia	Is a pale yellow gelatinous mass with a red border.
Herpes Sores	Are pancake shaped beige white pearly particles of energy.
I	
Inflammation	An active inflammatory disorder is indicated by a bright yellow white area whose edges define the parameters of the affected area. The outside edges of an inflamed area further describe what is occurring: An active inflamed edge is red. An inflamed edge that is growing or spreading is in a multidimensional flame or zigzag shape with an inner clear red energy surrounded by a yellow orange exterior edge. A green edge is an area in which physical restoration has begun.
Infection	The amount of gold orange energy over an area represents the degree of infection; red edges determine how invasive the infection has penetrated that region.
Intestines	Healthy intestines have a shiny finish, while inflamed intestines have a matt grey blue finish.(Chrome vs. stainless)
Intestines Peritoneal Sack	An inflamed peritoneum sack looks like a swollen thickness of about ¼

	inch and is a grey burgundy. You can see the healthy intestine inside of the sack as a separate energy slide.
Intermittent Energy	Intermittent energy shows up as flickering on and off. The length of timing between flickering determines how often the health issue event comes and goes.
IV Ports	Appear as a shiny silver object shaped and sized like a port and residing under the skin in the area that they were placed.
J	
Jock Itch	Is a motley red rash slice encased in a pale yellow pasty shell slide.
Joint Pain	Presents as a muddy overlay over the joint affected and lights up if its initial arthritis. It is also spiked with purple blue which determines the amount of pain.
K	
Kidney, Bleeding	Has a thick almond colored exterior shell that is lined with slices of bright red vertical striated bars.
Kidney, Dysfunction	The affected area looks very dark navy blue with spots of black; however the outermost edge of the entire energy slide is chocolate brown.
L	
Leg Cramps	Create a pale gold overlay on the muscle with a purple blue flame edge. The height of the flame determines the degree of cramping.

Leukemia	Leukemia looks like bright white running/traveling Christmas lights throughout the entire body's vascular system and is prevalent in all of the viewing areas. To further analyze what is going on in a specific segment of the body, you must ask to dismiss this screen since it will permeate all energy slides.
Lip Biting Inside of	There will be a dark edge that looks like an inverted comb that runs along the outside edge line of the affected lip.
Liver Alcoholism	A liver that is still functioning and yet affected by alcoholism will present an orchid colored edge where the liver tissue is being destroyed. The destroyed area will be burgundy black.
Liver Cirrhosis	See Cirrhosis

Load Bearing
     Energy
	Load bearing energy is a pale to dark chocolate brown over layer of energy in the direction of the weight bearing.
	     Ex: The outside of the left leg would have this layer if a person always favored standing on their left leg. A neck and shoulder area would have this energy overlay if the person tilted their head to the aforementioned side.

Lymph Nodes	Inflamed lymph nodes are yellow with an orange red tinged exterior. If the inflammation or infection is draining, the lymph drainage system

	looks like tree roots or tributaries extending from the main source.
Lungs Cancer	See Cancer
Lungs, Fluid in Lungs	Fluid filled lungs are a pale slate sky blue with a silver energy slice encapsulating the lung's exterior parameters.
Lungs, Fluid - Blood	This is a red burgundy soft jello like liquid energy that seeps from the inner lung lining, unless it's from a lung lesion or a specific area.
Lung Bleed Fluid Dissipation	Fluid filled lungs that is ongoing is a dark pasty pudding consistency blue black burgundy that heavily hangs over the lungs and doesn't shift on a slide.

Lungs
    Pneumonia
        Blue
        Cinnamon
	The outer layer is a heavy royal blue with the 2nd layer a bubbly deep cinnamon slate gray, all located *inside* the lung area.

Lungs
    Pulmonary
    Embolism
	A pulmonary embolism is a dark black tangled mass spot surrounded by a deep red edged burgundy where the actual clot is lodged. A charcoal gray mass/ area filters out around the initial dark mass and creates a second over layer energy slide that represents the physical energy area that is affected and non functioning due to that embolism. Each embolism, presents an individual energy slice in the surrounding tissue that is rendered non functional by that clot.

Lungs Smokers	This is a silver haze on the top level of viewing the lung's energy slide. The depth of the gray colored energy determines how much a person smokes.
M	
Medicine, Influence of	Medicine can be so strong that an entire energy area can be blacked out. If that is the case then the client should be advised that they may need to lower the dosage. Example: Paralysis client on too strong leg spasm meds disallowed any viewing of the spinal area.
Menstrual Cramps	This condition presents pulsating pale blue intermittent energy on top of a bulbous deep burgundy red energy slide overlaying the female reproductive area.
Menstrual Cycle	Pulsating red energy overlaying the area of the uterus. If the periods have heavy bleeding, the area will have a very heavy feel and a deep burgundy undertone.
Mitral Valve Sluggish	A mitral valve defect looks like a dragging purple blue dark grey energy slice that "sorta misses" formulation of an energy area. The energy will begin to form, and coagulate then it will dissipates and start the process over again.
Missing Organ	Is a black non electromagnetic area shaped like the original organ in the organ's location. If an organ never developed from birth, there won't

	even be an energy imprint.
Mole or Birthmark	Is a flat non dimensional area of black energy like a thin dime or whatever the exact parameters are.
Muscle Atrophy	Muscle atrophy has a prune like retracted and diminished cellular slice that also shows the original healthy energy slide in clear form superimposed over the atrophied zone.
Muscle, Hyper Extended	Shows a silken looking sheer silver stretched energy, (think stretched out panty hose), over the damaged part.
Muscle Strained or Sprained	White milky murky cloudy overlay of the muscle, tendon or ligament involved.
Muscle Weakness	The muscle energy area shows up then fades, repeatedly. It's thinner energy than healthy muscle tissue.
N	
Navel "In"	Looks like a chocolate brown inward scooped bowl.
Necrosis	Is a black space that is void of electromagnetic energy.
Nerves Neural Pathways	Tracking neural pathways is a beautiful site! Healthy functioning nerve pathways look like pale blue iridescent silken continuously connected delicate spider webbing. Broken pathways have jagged yellow purple blue misfiring ends or black nonfunctioning ends.

Nerve Damage	If a nerve is damaged it will show a navy blue dark disruption along the pale blue webbing.
Nerve Disconnection	A disconnected nerve will look like an erratic bright light, think sparks from a broken electrical circuit, at the point of disconnection.
Nerve Reconnection	To reconnect or regenerate a nerve's original function, you must overlay a new electromagnetic pathway around and over the original damaged nerve path, like putting electrical tape over and around broken or damaged electrical wiring.
Nose Broken	Splintered splattered black energy emanating from the area broken that has red edge fragments of bone or cartilage.
O	
Osteoarthritis	Swollen red boney spot energy, with an inner lining of pale blue and an outer lining of yellow.
Osteoporosis	Osteoporosis looks like pale blue lined sponge cream colored holes that represent energy that has "vacated" the normal energy mass within open areas within the affected bones.
Out of Body Energy	Out of body energy is usually seen in severe trauma, extreme pain, body function impairment situations or towards the end of life transition. Out of body energy looks like dark black "snow" (like on a television screen) over the physical body.

	If you are watching out of body energy and it begins to pulsate (i.e. throb), in a downward stacking manner, in colors of gold (immune system) and red (life force energy) and royal blue (if there is severe pain) that pattern usually means the soul is returning into the body. As you watch, the black "snow" will become less and transmute into the original shape and specific physical energy of the area that you were previously viewing.
	If the soul is deciding **if** they want to stay, the black snow energy will appear constant while they are making their choice and then revert back to physical energy if they stay. If you have been retained to view a client and you cannot "find/ read" anything but black snow energy, I suggest you inform the client that the individual you are viewing is making life choices.
	If you review the energy at a later time period, and find a renewed physical energy image, the soul has chosen to remain on earth a while longer.
	If the individual is in the process of life force transition, black snow will incrementally increase and turn into swirling violet purple flecks from the start of the process usually 24 – 48 hours prior to their total transition and will never revert back to physical energy.
Ovaries Fibrosis	The interior of the ovary will look like fine gauge knotty tangled steel wool. You can discern by looking at the

	"steel wool areas" exactly where the most of the fibrous areas are.
P	
Pain Patterns	Red in an inverted v pattern pointing inwards towards the area means the pain is created from outside pressure. Blue emanating outward for the area means the pain is from the area itself. Blue purplish white created outside of any area is generated by nerve stimulated pain impulses. Phantom pain is in this last category.
Pancreatic Polyps	Look like little pink hedgehogs embedded in the pancreatic wall.
Paralysis	Paralysis creates a sheer pale blue wispy color over the affected area. If the energy image is intermittent (i.e. comes and goes) it is inconsistent paralysis as in MS onset and then remission. The paralysis is permanent if the pale blue area is integrated into the bioenergy field. Transient event generated paralysis is represented by a pale blue layer that shifts and disappears on top of the affected area as you pass through the age layers of the client's energy.
Parkinson's Leg Stiffening	Shows up as vertical red energy bars moving up and down constantly overlaying the area that has arrested movement
Pituitary Tumor	Is a secretive little floating dark navy mass that hovers over the origination

	site of black. This tumor usually shows up from the back, side or top of head or up from under the throat position.

Precursor Energy Future	Precursor energy comes before a medical issue totally enters into the human energy field and often illuminates an energy pattern that potentially will lead to the development of another health issue or condition.
	
	    Precursor energy or future energy is much thinner and more delicate than dense human energy field. It is in the furthest layer outside the physical field as it has not yet occurred.
	
	    Example: Cystitis will hover over and engulf the area of the bladder in which it will occur. Cancer metastasis will appear as a white film over the body area in which it will be identified. I had a cancer client that I said would have kidney cancer at the urethra. The precursor energy took 1.5 years to penetrate the human energy field enough for a MRI to detect the affected area.
	
	    Another client's precursor energy indicated that he was going to have a heart attack. He could have prevented this energy from descending into his physical realm with lifestyle changes. He did not, and had to have a quadruple bypass 2.5 years later.
	
	    Even upcoming sore throats, flu etc show up in this manner.

Psychic Energy	Burns out around the edges of the

	area you are looking at like a fire, or shows up as a dark grey stain in brain matter.
Pulsating Anything	A red energy that looks like a large comma that pulsates over the area i.e. goes to a point then pulsates into a fat oval then drops back to the original shape then repeats over and over demonstrates the energy viewed is throbbing from blood, pain, electromagnetic dysfunction, infection, etc.
R	
Radiation Energy	Is a scarlet red and a completely separate layer from the human energy field. It retains the particular shape of the object that delivers the radioactive energy and fits over the physical energy that you are viewing. Example: Radiation energy for a brain tumor immolates the helmet shape that is used to deliver the radiation to the patient's skull. Radiation for a spinal tumor, delivered in front of the ribcage looks like a large yet see through 4 inch thick circular disc (i.e. the area covered by the radiation beam) fitting above the patient's physical energy field.
Rectal Immobility Anal Opening	Anal openings that lack the elasticity to expand and contract normally look like a medium grey PVC pipe over the area that has lost its motility, rather than flexible cording.
Rheumatoid Arthritis	Is a blue gnarly red burgundy energy stuck around and onto the disturbed

	sections.

Ribs,
    Bruised
        Blue purple
        Black
        Deep red
        Rib
	Black spots designate the point of impact with deep red energy encapsulating the bruised rib area. A blue and purple overlay is visible if extreme pain is associated with the bruising.

Root Canal	Shows up as a bright white edged in yellow vertical image under the tooth that is affected
Rosecea	Pulsating red blotches overlaying the subcutaneous skin cells in the affected areas. Rosecea is different than skin blotching energy because it is actively pulsating rather than being a dormant overlay.
Runny Nose	Light pale beige- spraying out of nose on side most affected.
S	
Scar Tissue	Scar tissue looks like a solid black mass due to the fact that no electromagnetic energy exists in those cells.
Scar Tissue Stretched	Scar tissue that has been stretched and creating pain will look like a pulled out brillo pad with a slice of golden fused overlay to indicate inflammation. If there is pain associated with this hyper extended scar tissue then there is a slice of blue over those two layers. Plastic surgery scars have a smooth look, due to the stitch feathering. When they are pulled, it looks like the

	consistency of spread out honey in a slate gray golden smear.
Sciatica	The slide begins at the point of origin in the lower back and burns red slices down the leg with a purple blue overtone.
Scrotum Undeveloped	A non developed scrotum is blank physical energy overlaid with a solid brown paste.
Scoliosis	Appears as a full pale grey overlay from the base of the neck to the bottom of the hips and is in the initial overview slide in a back scan. To illustrate when the misalignment is, the apex vertebras (example T3 and T7) will light up to indicate and initiate the gray area that then extends down to the lower lightened vertebrae which indicates the bottom of the scoliosis area.
Seizures	Look like bursts of purple light with red and yellow edges of purple pointed flares.
Shingles	Is an eggshell patch(s) with royal blue edges.
Sinus problems	Light up inside the sinus cavities, and then present what is wrong: Golden sinuses are infected, blue is painful, and red is bleeding.
Skin Poor Circulation	Poor circulation appears as rust colored areas hovering over the area of the skin. As the lack of circulation progresses to no circulation that area becomes more and more blue black.

Slipped Disc	A slipped disc looks like a bowl of cream beige lined by black spilt jello pudding, oozing to the dislocated side.
Slumping	Pronounced forward slumping or rounded shoulders shows up as a heavy dark brownish gray area between the pectoral muscles, and shows the compressions into the inner body cavity's energy field.
Smell, Loss of	A thin solid black overlay at the end of the nose covering each affected nostril and extending back about ½ inches into the nose structure.
Smoking	Coats the lungs in shear veils of pale grey energy. The longer the smoking, the deeper the layers of gauze grey.
Sore Throat	Gray hovering mass surrounding the neck.
Sores	Are white pock mark holes in the healthy skin energy.
Spasms Continuous	Are jerky green gray energy that rolls like a jump rope, bearing down, then lifting, then down and lifting. The second slide of energy will determine what causes the spasmodic condition.
Sphincter muscle	See Rectum
Spinal curvature	See Scoliosis
Spinal fluid	Appears as liquid iridescent cellophane.

Spleen 　Swollen	White puffy white blobs over the image of the normal spleen area.
Stent or Port	Looks like shiny highly reflective chrome like surface. Some ports may appear to be fuzzy pale white plastic usually with an inflamed area surrounding the site. 　A scar tissue from a port will show up in the past energy as a port and then fade to a dark black no active area for the final scar when the port has been removed.
Stitches	Normal Stitches present as pale gray strips or hyphenations, unless surgical glue was included which will look like waded up old dried chewing gum. 　Example: If the client has intestinal stitches, then they will show up on the outside of the colon. Any scar tissue or aberrations of the skin involved in the sutures will show up on the inside of the area. 　FYI- If there is a blockage of the colon due to that scar tissue of "clumped gathered" skin from a resection, check to see it could be interfering with bowel movement. 　Feathered stitches look like escalator stripes integrated between the original spaces.
Stomach, Gastric Bypass Surgery	Shows the cut area and the bands around the remaining tissue, plain and simple!
Stomach Spasms 　Cramps	Appear as a medium blue pulsating spiking starburst slice overlaying the stomach or small intestine areas that

	is affected. The amount of pulsating will alert you to the frequency of spasm activity.
Stroke	Stroke shows up as navy where the damage is, and all the vascular systems involved are either shriveled or exploded.
Sty	Bright green red encapsulated in gold white surrounded by pink on the eye.
T	
Teeth Crowns	Teeth that are crowned have a blackened root area, a pale glowing base and a slate gray tooth image at the crown site.
Testicles Jock Itch	Testicles that have a rash have a red amber color over them that are then overlaid with a slice of pale yellow film indicating a current and active inflammation.
Thoracic Vertebral Fracture	All vertebrae fractures look like thick blue black lines. Thoracic vertebrae are deeper in the body than cervical or lumbar, and have more muscle energy overlay that you need to move over to view them correctly.
Throat Drainage	Pale streaks of iridescent silver overlaying the affected esophagus.
Tinnitus	A pale sliver of a vibrating highly refined incredibly fast lightened area in the inner ear midway along the tube. About ¼ inch long.
Transition MIDI while in	As I appraised a client's energy something concerned me. Although

Transition	her "spirit" would take the energy I sent to view her body, her body never brightened. It was if her body was not participating, vacating and not responding to show me her energy.
	Most bodies look solid. Her energy was like looking through layers of mesh or very fine screen wire. It was not a solid form.
	When I have seen this with a client's response, that client's body was not long here on this earth.
	Prediction wise, I cannot give an accurate timetable of physical energy that is hard to see. NOT from a "can't get to it to view", but from a "not all of it is here to see" perspective. You ask yourself: Where did the scattered energy go??? Where is the physical energy that should be a solid form?
	Usually in a situation like this, a part of the client's life force energy has started the transition process.
	If the client during this time has dreams about those from the other side or sees or hears from people that are deceased, the answer to these questions is a STRONG indicator of the transition timeframe, or that the client is in "transition mode."
	This energy variability usually begins several months out and increases as departure time nears.
Thyroid	Hypothyroidism shows energy that pulsates upward from the thyroid, Hyperthyroidism defines energy wave patterns that flow down and away from the thyroid.
Thyroid	A large peach colored fuzzy overlay

Irradiated	hovers atop the thyroid that has received radiation treatment.
Tissue Removed in Surgery	Tissue that has been removed in a surgical procedure still appears in the bioenergy field. It looks like a clear bag overlaying, encapsulating and in the exact same place the original tissue inhabited.
TMJ	Is a bright purple blue triangle over the lower "L" of the jaw area, with brushed streaking energy up the side of the face.
Toes with Reynaud's	Glow red with a beige heavy cream encapsulation around them.
Toenail Damage Fungus	White cloudy shapes over the affected area. Fungus has a murky pale yellow mustard paste coloration.
Tongue Coated	A coated tongue appears as a pale murky gray jellyfish like a gelatinous blob floating over the area involved.
Transition Energy	Is counter clockwise swirling royal purple energy that is moving very slowly and going upward as the physical body detaches itself from the eternal life force energy. The purple swirls overlays the entire physical body which looks like a very diffuse black screen netting. It's as if the human energy field within the body is perforated with myriad micrometer holes. The energy that is missing from the body's energy's holes has already transitioned into another form on the other side.

U	
Ulcers	Are deep burgundy red with an overlay of inflamed yellow. With a scalloped edge

Urination
   Post Urination
   Drip
	At the exterior opening of the bladder, a very thin pale blue gray overlay of energy pools at that opening and remains in position. The energy will flash off and on until you recognize the symptom.

Uterus, Biopsied	A biopsied section looks like a flat dark gray slate area with a red puncture hole.
Uterus, DNC	The uterine lining will have a slate gray rimmed area of cells next to the inside currently functioning tissue.
V	
Vaginitis	Vaginitis presents as a dull pale beige overlaid with a thin film of the palest iridescent gray, delineating the drainage area.
Varicose Veins	Varicose veins look like blue purple bruises over the normal leg.
W	
Weighted Energy	This energy can be felt and appears visually heavier than the surrounding energy. It can denote whether a person tilts their head to one side of the other, leans left or right, and walks with the load bearing weight on one side of the leg or foot etc. This describes the sensation of what the

	energy is producing or doing. Like a lean to the left in the posture that is created by scoliosis.
Whiplash	Looks like pulsating spiraling rocking back and forth pale red burgundy energy in the involved cervical vertebrae.
Wisdom Tooth Removed	Shows as a black area where the root used to inhabit the jawbone.

In Conclusion:

One question that I get frequently is:
Is it possible to say "show me what acne looks like" and be able to "see" acne without a client?
Answer: YES

All I do is request the disease or disorder, and then the generic image that appears in my mind's eye/vision.

In addition to the verbal images in my upcoming Encyclopedia, I plan to provide illustrations of the energy patterns that I describe.

My Website www.BrentAtwater.com has a section of my Paintings that Heal®. These paintings represent exactly what I see as the generic disorder's initial energy pattern.

Then I paint the energy that is needed to heal that disease over the first layer.   See what you think.

All other integrative medicine fields have a resource reference. This is my Gift to further facilitate YOUR Gifts!

If you like, email us and we'll put you on the
"reserve an encyclopedia for me" list, or
come to or host an event for one of our presentations.
Brent@BrentAtwater.com

Part 4

Detach, remove and release from
your client and session.
Go onto
your next experience
unfettered and unaffected by
energy, issues or entities.

Animal Medical Intuitive Diagnostic Imaging™
AMIDI

To me, pets are beloved family members, thus a short section on working with them My AMIDI book will be released in 2011.

Prior to the Appointment

I have my animal parents fill out the same forms for their pets. I suggest that you do the same because you are under the same legalities while working on an animal.

Animal Energy Frequencies

Do not lower your energy frequency to go down to an animal's health frequency and vibrational range while communicating, viewing or healing.

An animal has a lower frequency range than your human energy field. You can acquire a massive headache dealing in their lowered energy realms. Set your intent to allow the energy that flows thru you to connect with and view the animal's energy.

Client Permission

A pet is used to human contact so they will usually not reject your work with them. However, like a human client, you must ask their permission to work with their energy.

I had a cat named Nikki, who said "no!" when I asked to work with him. It took a great deal of negotiating. He was angry with the veterinarian for feeling lousy. I had to promise him that his kidneys would be better and he would no longer hurt before he allowed me to work with him.

To this very day, when I call and talk with his person on the phone, he recognizes my energy and will come to the phone and hang around just purring.

Abused, Defensive or Feral Animals

Do not be defensive when approaching this category of animals! Set your intent, acknowledge their existence,
State: I come in peace and mean no harm. I you want to help you, may I have permission to do so.

If they refuse, you must honor that fact.

Ask if you may work with them on site, or by distance. If they decline, send them energy **"to use as they so choose"** so they may use your Gift any way they want.

Animals in Transition

Prior to transition 24 to 48 hours before crossing over a human and pet begin pulling in their energy field. If you can't find a client's energy they may be preparing to cross.

Ask the animal if it wants to cross.

Ask their owner to ask in their heart to confirm.

Ask the animal if it wants help crossing.

Ask what kind of help it wants.

Give the animal permission to leave and to do what it needs to do for its highest and best good and don't perform your scan.

Preparing for a MIDI Session with Animals

First clear the animals by removing any old energy or entities.

Place a bubble/cocoon around them to keep them shielded and feeling safe. Create that bubble around your client by using the shielding prayer. It holds their heart and soul in love and stabilizes and calms them while you work.

Use the same quadrant sectioning and same procedures that you use in a human MIDI with the exception of using a veterinarian's anatomy guide for concepts and verbiage with each animal- dog, cat, and horse.

And of course, it's "show me what I need to see and tell me what I need to know." Ask ask Ask!

The Universe is the library of "all" knowledge and directions on how to do anything! Ask, even Ask why no answer. Ask, Show me what to do. Just ask, every answer for everything is available!

Basically, you conduct an animal MIDI like that of a human except you do not go down to their frequency level. Use all of the other human input methods for my animal intuitive diagnosises also.

A cumulative "for the records" summary is always a great idea, perhaps with a drawing locating the issues

I suggest that you work with your animal clients one day and human clients on another day. It will make viewing easier for you because you will not be sorting through, interchanging and interfacing multiple frequency range levels.

Business Details

Attitude

There is no competition. The Universe sends you the exact clients for your special Gifts in correct timing. If you need to persuade a client to work with you that is not a good sign because you have already tainted the purity of the energy exchange.

Value Your Gift

Your Gift is just that. Do not devalue your ability for fear of losing business.

Certification of Your Gift!

Should I have certification and lots of degrees from all the masters & teachers? Your choice! I am certified by God and client results!

In the middle of the night I received a frantic call from a friend desperate for help for one of her best girlfriends who was admitted to the hospital on a ventilator due to fluid accumulation in her cancerous lungs and wasn't expected to live till morning.

I agreed to help her. I did a MIDI and did energy work all night. By dawn she had stabilized and was being weaned from the ventilator. Her doctors were floored and had never thought results of this nature were possible.

Several days later when Best Friend was able to talk, she called and thanked me and said she wanted me to meet and work with her doctor who was with Sloan Kettering.

When I spoke with her doctor on the phone at her insistence and introduction the conversation went like this:

D: "Tell me Ms Atwater, what IS it you do?"
B: "I say my prayers, set my intent, focus, watt up and send
    healing energy to my client to facilitate the desired results."

D: "And where did you get your medical training?"
B: "I have none."

D: "Where did you study medicine?"
B: "I have never studied medicine."

D: "And where do you get your information"

B: "From the voices in my head."

D: "Lets' see, you have never studied medicine, have no
    medical training, and get your information from 'voices in
    your head', is that correct?"
B: "yes Sir"

D: "Who do you think you are, interfering in my patients' life
    and why do you even think you can help her?"
B: "Because of her results."

D: "You leave my patient alone!"
B: "No sir, She's hired me to facilitate her healing!"

And so certification goes!!!

Training and Certification

Does having 24 certificates on the wall make you feel better or more secure? If it does, by all means go get several. I think that the various approaches and methods and theories of healing modalities are absolutely wonderful IF they ignite in your soul, your remembrance of what you can innately contribute or activate new dimensions of your abilities to benefit others.

However, never doubt that you, like I, might be in the "just do it" Club (as the Nike ad says). It's the benefits and results your client receives that matters most, not framed degrees and certifications.

Professional Behavior

A lot of beginning practitioners will answer the phone any hour of the day or night on any day of the week, and then complain about their client base. Set parameters of what you want: Clientele, office hours, et al. Value what you do so others will.

If you don't value your time, neither will someone else. And anyone will take a free sample. Ask to bring in the type of client that you think that you want. Then you can determine if it's truly your direction. Sometimes a multitude of multi tiered directions are part of expanding your journey and not the specific end of your trip.

I incorporated my business under the suggestion of my Father who is an attorney. He also worded portions of my consent forms that are in this book. In today's world, as sad as it may be; there are individuals who will try to sue for no apparent reason when you have worked on them in good faith. If you are incorporated, then your personal losses should be less, if the "business" is sued.

I am always amused by alternative practitioners who wave goodbye while saying "Love and Light" when leaving. Can you imagine Carolyn Myss saying that to a neurosurgeon after leaving intensive care? You get my point!

If you want to be treated as a professional you have to be one!

Privacy

Under no circumstances are you allowed to give client names or health circumstances, unless you have it in writing that you have permission to relate their "story." Your work with each client is confidential!

What do I charge for my services since I don't think I know what I'm doing?

Ask your guides, the Gift will unfold thru you and your guidance will tell you what to charge all along the way.

I was "told" to start at $185.00, why those figures- I have no idea. I had lots of clients. Then I decided to lower it to "help" folks. I lost client volume. When I went back to work for $185.00, the onset of those seeking my help began again.

No fee schedule determines your greatness! You will get the exact client in the exact financial bracket that you came to serve! Think Mother Theresa. Even Oprah helps in healing others by expanding awareness. Healers come in all forms and financial strata. No one is more important than the other. It's just their assignment level in this incarnation. If your clients are falling off, then even reassess your fee scale. The Universe has a way of redirecting your course if you're not on track. How can the Universe help you, if YOU stand in the way???

Billing

It is my practice for a client to fill out a contract prior to our appointment. It insures that the client is serious about our appointment, and even includes a forfeiture clause should the client be unable to notify my office that they need to reschedule. I believe as a single practitioner, this is a solid foundation investment for your business exchange and booking time.

Payment

Always create an exchange that has a full circle of balance. You are paid money or receive a barter presentation as the top half of the circle. Then you give back to the payee your services in exchange for what you received. **U** This completes the bottom half of the circle. The transaction is then balanced. **O**

If you give things away "free," i.e. the receivee just walks away and hopefully says thanks, then that transaction has a Karmic debt of "owing" and is unbalanced, no matter how much "good" you think you did.

Many healers think "giving away with love" is "doing good." That thought is partially correct. Oftentimes the "givor "feels empty inside, depleted of resources and unfulfilled. That is a correct emotional response because ANY balanced interchange in life must have giving AND receiving which is activated and regenerated from the giving. One sided transactions are unbalanced and open Karmic debt.

Appointment Payment

Due to the fact that I work internationally, I require my clients to pay for their appointment in order to secure a place in my schedule. Sadly, before I adopted that practice, I had many that "promised to pay" the other half at the end of the appointment or for the sliding fee on a monthly basis and never did. I allow their credit card payments be their monthly remittance for our session.

Sliding Scale Fee

If it is your choice to present a sliding scale fee, that's great. I do not find it appropriate for my client base. Over the years I have found that when people ask for a discount, it later becomes apparent in other conversations that they have spent "thousands" with doctors and other practitioners, so this has made me very wary.

You can't imagine the stories that I have heard about why someone can't pay. I politely inform them that while I appreciate their candor and understand a budget, when their financial situation changes we'll make an appointment.

My heart chooses the recipients of my pro bono work in hospitals, with veterinarians, rescue leagues and just plain folks.

Discounts and "Specials"

A lot of practitioners give "free" sessions in order to lure business. Almost everyone will take a free sample of almost anything. Renowned physicians do not have to give free consultations or surgeries. Your reputation for accuracy, knowledge and integrity will bring clients to you. Advertising "freebies" looks like you need to attract clients for your work.

I prefer to stand in knowledge and Trust that I get exactly who I'm supposed to work with and when, rather than "hawk my wares."

Many practitioners also give volume or bulk discount rates. Have you ever heard of a hospital MRI, x ray or CT scan technician say "since we have viewed this area in your body on multiple occasions, we are going to give you a discount"? To me, if you have a strong practice, you are undermining your work. Potential clients will wait until you are having a "special," or will always be asking for a "discount."

Do you think Carolyn Myss, Louise Hayes, Judith Orloff, Donna Eden, Deepak Chopra, Dr. Oz or whomever you think is "the" personality in your energy medicine or intuitive healing or intuitive development world would give Freebies or discounts? Even *"The Secret"* crowd would just set their intent and manifest business. Deliberate pro bono work yes, charitable contributions yes, educational materials yes, presentations at learning centers yes, etc.

When in doubt ask yourself, how would your favorite professional handle this?

Have you ever heard a person going into the emergency room, MRI or asking their dentist, "Will you perform your services for less?" *after* they have scheduled the appointment? Hard times may necessitate this question. In my opinion, it's disrespectful to the holistic and integrative medicine community. If necessary, clients should ask if you will lower your fees for their situation *before* a session and not prey on your "love" based profession.

Too many desperate "freebies" and "discounts" have created this atmosphere. I understand helping those under financial duress, we've all been there. However, "because it's a "Gift" and "you work from Love" doesn't pay the bills. Frustrated and strapped "healers" filled with "joy" AND underlying stress, need to rethink and revaluate their work ethics. Even ministers are paid salaries by the Church as are the Pope, the Rabbis, etc... So being compensated at a professional level for professional services represents alternative therapies, to me, better than discounting the Gifts that God / the Universe gave to you to benefit others!

I believe that atmosphere has also created another mindset- that alternative practitioners will take whatever they can get during *any hour of the day or night* to try to "prove" their worth or "giving for love." No parameters create no respect!

In the allopathic world, you go to the physician that your budget and or insurance, network or circumstances necessitates, and there is no "discussion" prior to your appointment re fees. You accept the billing of the healthcare provider that you have chosen, or you search for one that offers the services you need in your price range.

Bartering

Many alternative therapists barter with each other exchanging services. This appears to be a common practice; however, I do not feel that this promotes professionalism. When I have been to conferences and as a keynote speaker, many individuals come up to me and ask "would you just take a quick look at me?" I say sure, contact me after the event is over.

When they contact me I treat them just like a client and have them fill out the forms and make payment. This may sound harsh; and it makes a lot of those folks a bit miffed, however during the same time I would be doing a "Freebie," I could be helping an individual resolve their health issues which would contributes to me paying my physician's bill. Most traditional medical personnel do offer a percentage off "to other doctors or professional equals and their immediate family." I feel that trade practice acknowledges real world finances AND professional respect.

I also receive an extraordinary amount of practitioners emailing me asking how to work with their energy, do a treatment for their client and a range of assorted questions about their personal energy work, practice et al.

Maybe I've been sequestered my entire life, but questions are asked in an educational setting. To me, you go to med school to ask the doctors questions, I also presume you'd take a class if you wanted that information. DO they ever think about the time it takes to write a detailed answer to their question, and that you might want a personal life outside of your appointment, speaking, writing or workshop schedule?

The parameters I mention above, I base on professional healthcare standards. To me, just because you work for God / the Universe, and God is love, you just don't walk around giving away what you are the steward of and complaining that you can't make a living and pay your bills.

Charitable Donations

If you want to give away your expertise, I suggest that you do it in a professional manner. Set aside a special timeframe or day for pro bono work. You can inform your client base or advertise that day as your "give back" day. Then keep a list of the clients, what services you provided, with a dollar amount affixed to each service and give that to your accountant at the end of the year as your charitable contributions/ donations. Or join an all volunteer health help organization like Volunteers in Medicine or donate your time and talents to local clinics and healthcare facilities.

Emergency Paperwork
The emergency room requires that you or someone with you fills out paperwork for the triage nurse and hospital records. I suggest your office require those forms also. Emergency situations should not negate paperwork! Those promising to "call back and give you their information," sadly, are not always reliable to do so. It took my heart about 10+ years to learn that!

Death
When your client becomes deceased, you do not owe a refund. Both the hospital and the doctors that treated the patient will send charges that were incurred up to the time of death. It is my suggestion that as a professional, do not dismiss your charges by "being nice" just because the client died. Health care facilities don't give death discounts. Death is a part of the cycle of life.

In Summary
I spend a lot of time working for free in veterinarian clinics, nursing homes, hospitals and private consultations. Often times I'll extend my services and hours way beyond what the client has purchased to help them get on tract. I don't advertise it. My heart tells me who and how to help, let yours do the same.

To keep your practice on track with email, contacts, phone calls, letters, et al interviews etc.
Every morning before you get out of bed...
State: God, I ask and it is my intent that you send to me today all those that would benefit from my products and services that will be for their highest and best good and those that would benefit me. Send them to me without delay so that I may serve You thru my work. Stop any and everything that interferes and impedes my progress. Thank you, Amen.
THIS ONE REALLY WORKS!!!!!!!

Websites If you have a website, I believe that you should publish your rates. A lot of practitioners do not publish their fees, so they can maneuver costs after they receive potential client information. To me, its professional ethics to state your charges up front like the traditional medical community does. Be proud of your fees whatever they are.

Website Disclaimers
The following is a standard Disclaimer.
THIS WEBSITE IS FOR INFORMATIONAL AND ENTERTAINMENT PURPOSES ONLY AND IS NOT A SUBSTITUTE FOR MEDICAL ADVICE, DIAGNOSIS OR TREATMENT.
For your protection, be sure that you display it where is can be prominently seen on your site. Other medical disclaimers should be displayed also.

"Learning Opportunity" Stories

"Don't touch her, she could give you energy"
I maintain a home in a small resort town. A lady had seen me work with her best friend who had come to me with 4th stage breast cancer. After our work together she is in remission.

While in the garden department of Wal-Mart, buying my spring flowers, I saw this lady and spoke to her. I was going to shake the hand of the woman's husband when she ran and jerked my hand away from him, saying "don't touch her she could give you energy."

Lesson: Sometimes the Gift is perceived by others incorrectly.
Hold fast to the good and benefits it does for others.

Use your talents wisely
After being on holiday, while unpacking my travel cases I twisted, bent down and tried to lift my hanging bag. I later learned that in the medical community that movement is called torque.

I fell on the floor while hearing a crunch and couldn't get up. I was delivered to the emergency room on a spinal board.

After pelvic x-rays the physician said they saw nothing. Having the Gifts that I do, I was able to look at myself and see that L1, L3 and T10 were fractured! I mentioned to the doctor that I wanted an MRI and that I wanted a thoracic x-ray. He complied with a lumbar MRI and suggested that I might have a slight fracture at L1.

I even have to take care of myself within the medical community, so I sought and found another leading healthcare facility that had more advanced equipment and that MRIed the images from the perspectives that I requested.

The images showed my fractures. My physicians prescribed the appropriate traditional medications and treatments. I added my alternative therapies.

Lesson: When you know your Gift has provided accurate information, use and present it wisely to help navigate those who don't have your expanded awareness. I believe that Integrative medicine is the best combination for the client!

First time seeing a shunt

My very first MIDI paying client was a wonderful family who had heard about my reputation for accuracy through one of the top 5 USA hospital's medical doctors.

I was nervous. I explained to them that this was my first time charging for my services. I hoped they would allow me to work, then give questions and then pay me if they thought the reading was "worth it."

I received every detail on target, except for the shiny straw thing in the liver that showed up in a sweeping 360 degree view. I had No idea what that as, and I asked, asked and asked so I wouldn't be embarrassed at not knowing.

 I asked them not to tell me what I was searching for so I could figure it out.

I finally heard "shunt." It was a bile duct shunt. My clients confirmed this fact and then paid me more than my fees for "caring enough to work so hard at being thorough."

Lesson: Don't be afraid of saying I don't know and let me figure it out! You need to give the Universe ample time to orchestrate all the viewing details and provide the words for your knowledge.

How I learned the distant viewing and healing was real.

A friend in Washington DC on one of the presidential committees asked me for a favor. He said it would be good representation for alternative energy healing (if I could do it).

I agreed and was contacted by a young lady in Germany, who was born with seizures on an ongoing daily basis. They were so prevalent that her life was completely controlled and consumed by watching her mediations and seizure schedule. She even had a wonderful seizure dog named Verde (which ironically means truth) who lived with and protected her.

We set the appointed time for me to work with her.
She called; I said my prayers, did a MIDI and then sent healing energy.

I requested that she let me know how the effects were and if there was anything unusual. The next day she phoned and stated her seizures had lessened. However it was most interesting that Verde was pushing the hospital's seizure alert button the entire time we were working together. Her boyfriend had to lock Verde in the bathroom.

During our second energy session, I asked that the alert unit be unplugged and Verde be left in the room while we were working. Again, true to his training Verde continuously pushed the hospital alert system with his paw indicating that he sensed unfamiliar and extra energy around his owner.

She called to thank me and tell me that her seizures had diminished down to only about one per day, and that she and her boyfriend were going on holiday for the first time in her life! Then I explained Verde's behavior was consistent with registering my energy while I was working with her. I wished her safe and happy travels and have received several other happy emails over the years.

Humans regretfully can "fake" a situation to their benefit. A dog, half a world away, will not fake sensing intense and abundant energy around his owner. Verde was acknowledging my energy surrounding and affecting his master.

Lesson: Verde taught me that I can focus my intent and direct palpable energy to a client across the globe. I never disputed distant MIDIs or healing energy again.

Child with steel rods in her spine

Seeking to have her child walk again, a Mother and I worked together for several sessions with a positive outcome.

When I was completing my MIDI, I would see shiny "straws" down the side of the child's vertebrae, then it would go away and then it would repeat itself. Having never seen this before, I explained that it looked like her child would be paralyzed, then healthy, and then paralyzed again according to the energy slides, with these "things" going down her back. I had no information on what "they" were.

The Mother then explained that her child had been paralyzed when she had steel rods inserted in her spine twice in an effort to stabilize her spine to help her walk. The insertions had created the times she was paralyzed, and had to be removed.

Lesson: It's not a crime to not be familiar with everything! Provide all of the details that you do know, and ask your client for assistance on the rest. Remember, even the traditional medical community is not perfect nor can provide 100% reliable or accurate information diagnosis or prognosis all the time.

Intuition by Permission only

While visiting a male friend's family at their beach residence, I would see him in the distance stop and catch his breath. This was a robust and hail hearty fellow, so of course this symptom was never mentioned to me. I on the other hand, intuitively picked up each incidence with trepidation inside. However I did NOT tap into his energy to see what was going on.

On the front porch at sunset one evening, I casually asked if I could look into his body. With a cocktail under his belt he bellowed "sure……………." I did a quick scan and saw something that I needed to tell him. I decided to wait until the next morning after we all went for our bike ride.

I casually said, "Have you had your aortic valve checked recently?" He stated that he had JUST gotten his yearly physical and was pronounced fine. I told him that his valve was bad, and if he kept up his party hearty lifestyle including fried foods et al it could be a disaster in the making.

Being wary of what I do, I asked him to "humor" me and ask his doctor to recheck his aortic valve when he returned two weeks later for blood test results during his follow-up visit. Jim remarked that his physician did not find a problem with that valve during his initial visit and could not imagine how all the testing missed it. But he would "humor me" to "test" what I said.

Returning from his follow up visit, he greeted me rather pale and let me know that indeed there was a problem with his valve that had been missed in his annual checkup. After that Jim asked if I saw anything else and was more receptive to my remarks and was actually listening.

I told him that with his fried foods, "wine, women and song" lifestyle, he was going to have a heart attack and would need bypass

surgery in 2 years. He said "I'm going to live and enjoy my life."
I said "your choice." My visit was over and we each went our separate
ways checking in on one another along the way.

Several years later (2 to be exact), out of the blue, I received
an email from another friend. She said "I thought you might want to
know that Jim had an unexpected quadruple bypass yesterday." I had
forgotten my prognosis and told her I'd check in on him.

I asked why he had not let me know that he had had this
procedure. He replied "it was exactly one day shy of your 2 years
prediction." He told only his Mother "because I didn't want to hear you
tell me I told you so!"

Lesson: Never tap into a friend without permission. Each person
chooses their life path, no matter how much you would like to warn
them or make it easler for their path by your knowledge of their future
energy. Bless their choices, make no judgments and keep on loving
them the way they are.

Diverticulitis versus Cancer

One of my most interesting learning opportunities came from a
client who called from a hospital across the United States. She was
being scheduled for emergency surgery the next day after she became
stabilized.

She had previously collapsed with extreme low blood pressure
and had excruciating pain in her upper intestines.

She called to ask me to perform an emergency MIDI about her
situation. Her doctor and two specialist oncologists, two CAT scans,
various X-rays and a MRI determined that she had colon cancer.
Therefore the decision was made to remove a major part of her
intestines. Needless to say she was not real happy.

As I looked around, I told her that my take was entirely
different. I saw an area in her intestines in her past energy that
indicated she had experienced a major bout with Diverticulitis that had
left an infection pocket in her intestinal wall.

Her present energy indicated that the areas aforementioned
had burst due to the infection compromising the intestinal wall, and
blood vessels had ruptured which caused her extreme pain and the
immediate lowering of blood pressure.

The area I saw was 6.5 inches in length and looked like ground
hamburger meat with mayonnaise for the infection and inflammation
area.

Her future energy indicated that they would take our about 8 inches of intestines at that site, the initial 6.5 inches with a precautionary inch on each side for good measure.
The surgery would be under 2 hours and she would be fine!

She mentioned again that the finest oncologists and imagining technicians had assured her that they were correct in their diagnosis, and it would probably be a 6 hour operation. Her husband was prepared to sit it out in the waiting area. I told him otherwise, and to prepare to go home early.

Because I had worked with this client before, I said, "You can believe them or God." "But Brent" she said "they did all the tests and all the technical imaging; they're the top specialists in their field!"

I said "Welp, its God's information versus traditional medicine."

Needless to say, I paced the floor almost all night long, worrying for her and quite frankly that my information may have been incorrect even though I believed with my entire being that God / the Universe doesn't make mistakes. Or maybe like the other client she was not supposed to know.

The surgery time started and I began pacing the floor keeping busy doing laundry, dusting or whatever to pass the time.

About 1 hour 45 minutes into the time specified for her surgery, I get a call from her husband. My first thought is "how bad is it?" He then proceeds to say, "You're not going to believe this, but the doctor just walked out here in the waiting room to give me an update. He said she didn't have Cancer and that it was an infected ruptured diverticulitis area that looked like ground hamburger meat. He actually described it Brent, the exact way you had described it to us. I was shocked and thrilled at the same time. She's in the recovery room now and will be able to go home in a few days."

I said all the perfunctory niceties and promptly got off the phone.

Then after singing the "thank you song" and doing "my thank you dance," I went directly to my knees and said "yeah you, God!"

Score: God one, Doctors O

I never doubt, never ever.

Go home
and
enjoy your life on earth!

Are there any Questions from the Audience?

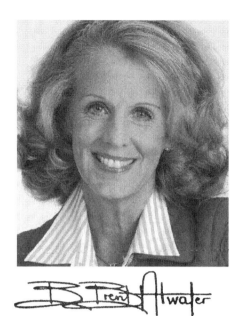

BRENT ATWATER
is a "Human MRI" and an internationally renowned medical intuitive, author, pet reincarnation authority, award winning artist, speaker and educator. www.BrentAtwater.com

At age 5 Duke University's Dr. J B Rhine, documented Brent's intuition during his initial study of ESP. After law school, Brent pioneered and founded MIDI, the field of Medical Intuitive Diagnostic Imaging™ the process of how to look inside a body to interpret bioenergy patterns that identify and diagnose past, current and future diseases and health issues.

Ms Atwater's leading edge work establishes evidence based research that creates and documents the bridging of traditional medicine and alternative therapies into holistic integrative medicine. Her client evaluations have documented, published and respected case results. www.BrentEnergyWork.com

In 1987 Brent founded the *Just Plain Love*® Charitable Trust to benefit children's and other worthwhile causes and later *Just Plain Love*® *Books.* As an Author she has released 10 books with more to follow. www.JustPlainLoveBooks.com (See list on last page)

Brent's Medical Intuitive books are groundbreaking resource books for holistic health, energy medicine, medical intuition, educators and other intuitive development and integrative health care professionals.

Always an animal lover, Ms Atwater pursued her pet reincarnation interest for 16+ years. Her research and the true stories gathered from around the world enabled Brent to describe the signs of pet reincarnation. She explains the phenomenal never-ending soul agreements and spiritual arrangements that create healing between you and your reincarnated animal companions in her 4 books on animal reincarnation.

As a medical intuitive Brent can see and predict future physical energy events therefore she can determine if and when your pet is going to reincarnate.

Ms. Atwater licensed her art and designs to the world's leading manufacturers and sold her highly sought after artwork to collectors from around the globe for 30+ years.

Brent is a pioneer in healing art medicine in the USA. In 2004 she produced the first pilot study that scientifically documented the healing energy, diagnostic abilities and healing benefits of her art for healthcare, *Paintings That Heal®*.

Brent is one of the contemporary American painters who are bringing forth a new cultural renaissance by integrating her classical artistic training with spirituality and directed energy infused into her art.

For the past 25 years, Brent has positively transformed and uplifted the lives of countless individuals and their beloved animal companions.

Ms Atwater's weekly radio shows, podcasts, audience participatory workshops, upbeat seminars, speaking tours and consultations are inspirational, educational and motivational.

Visit Brent on Twitter, Facebook, YouTube, MySpace, Tumbler, et al.

Visit www.BrentAtwater.com and www.JustPlainLoveBooks.com

The *Just Plain Love*® Story

"Experiencing a pediatric intensive care, oncology, burn or trauma unit to me, is a heart wrenching jolt to anyone's world. I had to summon all my "heart" to handle the various states of disrupted life. Right then and there I decided that a positive Light needed to shine on the hearts and minds of these struggling little souls, so new to earth and so old to the diseases, health issues and medical conditions whose very procedures and treatments ravaged their young bodies.

I decided that I was going to find a way to offer a "positive spin" on all of the health issue negatives and to create a portal of communication, and a treasure of heartwarming and reassuring perspectives to those "hands off" subjects.

Additionally I want to inspire a muffled laugh, instigate a tiny smile, mischievous giggle or just create an environmental change and safe place for even a brief moment that would add a sparkle to a weary eye.

AND I was going to give a comforting and supportive symbolic "hug" to each patient and reader by filling them with a sense of pride in themselves for having endured their own health battle and surrounding issues. Plus, I would provide a tangible and permanent way to honor and celebrate their courage!

I was unable to have children, so this is my way of giving back. In 1987 the Just Plain Love® Charitable Trust was born."

Brent Atwater's Other Dream:
Just Plain Love® Plays, Performances & Educational Programs for Children with "Poof" the Angel & "Friend" the pet angel therapy dog.

Surely, Ms Atwater dreams, there can be participatory mini skits/plays held in healthcare and medical facilities lasting about 5 to 15 minutes that would hold a patient's attention, entertain, educate, rehabilitate and provide a few safe moments of mental relief through laughter, plus providing each patient with a tangible Badge of Honor to reward and recognize their courage.

For the past 20+ years Brent Atwater has researched, tested, rewritten and reworked each children's healing book and play according to the storytelling responses and reactions from healthy and unhealthy readers, caregivers, family, friends, medical and healthcare professionals, clients and her storytelling audience.

Brent Atwater's dream is to inspire the creative imagination of readers of all ages to replace negative thoughts about health issues, medical experiences, rehabilitative therapy and reentry into society with a positive "spin" on their journey to health and well being.

Message to Book Clubs and Professional Associations and Organizations

I'd be delighted to speak with you over the phone or in person.

Please email me at

Brent@BrentAtwater.com

BrentAtwater@live.com

Just Plain Love® Books

inspiring thoughts that provide smiles, hugs and healing
for every reader's heart!

Other Just Plain Love® Titles
in Audio, EBooks, Hardcover, Kindle, and Paperback

Children's Books:
Cancer Kids—God's Special Children!
Cancer and MY Daddy

Holistic Integrative Energy Medicine, Intuitive Development:
Medical Intuition, Medical Intuitive Diagnosis, MIDI- Medical
Intuitive Diagnostic Imaging™ & AMIDI
Animal Medical Intuitive Diagnostic Imaging™
Encyclopedia of Bioenergy Patterns that Identify Disorders
AMIDI- Animal Intuitive Diagnosis

Health, Self Help /Healing, Mind Body Connection:
Healing Yourself! 23 Ways to Heal
Diseases, Disorders, Medical Conditions & Health Issues
How to Overcome Your Health Problems: Solutions for a Better
Quality of Life

Animal Lovers' Books:
the Dog with a "B" on His Bottom!   - A pet loss Gift book
Animal & Pet Reincarnation and Animal Communication
"I'm Home!" a Dog's Never Ending Love Story
"I'm Home!" a Cat's Never Ending Love Story
"I'm Home!" a Horse's Never Ending Love Story
Animal Reincarnation: Everything You Always Wanted to Know!

We hope you enjoyed this Just Plain Love® Book.
If you would like information about Just Plain Love® Books,
contact: Brent@BrentAtwater.com

Visit Brent Atwater's websites:
www.BrentAtwater.com
www.JustPlainLoveBooks.com
www.BrentEnergyWork.com

Made in the USA
Charleston, SC
02 March 2011